FROM PICKY TO POWERFUL

Other books by Maryann Jacobsen:

Fearless Feeding

The Family Dinner Solution

How to Raise a Mindful Eater

What Does Your Tummy Say?

FROM PICKY TO POWERFUL

The Mindset, Strategies and Know-How You Need to Empower Your Picky Eater

Maryann Jacobsen, MS, RD

DEDICATION

This book is dedicated to my blog readers. Every time I wrote about picky eating you responded. Thus, a book was born.

CONTENTS

Introduction

FROM GUILT TO GAINED PERSPECTIVE

Stephanie fed her baby a laundry list of foods to expose him to a wide variety of flavors at an early age: avocado, beets, lentils, barley, etc. She made almost all of her baby food, starting with veggies and adding sweet fruits later. Now he is two and would prefer to live off Dino nuggets and French fries. "If I had to sum it all up, I think we are disappointed that we did everything 'textbook' from the beginning and ended up with the same results as though we hadn't put in any effort," she said. "He won't eat veggies unless it's a potato, and he prefers to consume calories only at breakfast and snacks with maybe a few bites of lunch or dinner."

I hear this from parents all the time. They offered their children a variety of wholesome foods when they were babies, and the kids gobbled every bit of it up. But around the age of two (sometimes earlier, sometimes later), eating habits take a turn and parents are frustrated. This frustration turns to guilt as many think, "What am I doing wrong?"

The problem is not your child's eating; it's that you weren't prepared for this inevitable stage in his food journey. You've been told if you do everything right, employ certain strategies, and manipulate food variety, picky eating can be prevented. This not only adds to the needless guilt you feel, *it's flat-out wrong.*

Although you undoubtedly help shape your child's eating over the course of her childhood, there are real scientific reasons kids become more selective with food at toddlerhood (discussed in detail in Chapter 1). Picky eating is a mix of normal development, fluctuations in appetite, genetics, individual eating style, temperament, and yes, how and what is being served.

But I think the most hurtful message of all is that picky eating is a parent's fault, that something you did or didn't do was wrong, and other parents with kids who eat everything somehow got it right. Did you know that Michael Pollan, best-selling author and popular foodie, has a very picky son? And that many dietitians and chefs complain about feeding their picky kids? According to one study, nearly half of children are picky at some point during early childhood.[1]

I'm here to tell you that picky eating is not only not your fault, it can be a rewarding experience if you change your perspective. In the groundbreaking book, *Raising Your Spirited Child,* Mary Sheedy Kurcinka helps parents view what society labels as "difficult children" in a positive light.[2] Many of the traits of the spirited child, like determination, are qualities that are an asset in adulthood; the secret is learning how to manage these strong personalities during childhood. The same holds true for picky eating.

Let's look at the positive aspects of picky eating for a moment. Who was more likely to survive in hunter-gatherer times when there were toxic plants around? Would it be the child afraid to eat unfamiliar food or the child who eats anything? Of course, it was the cautious kid. And what adult wouldn't benefit from eating small amounts at dinner if they simply weren't hungry? Picky kids don't eat more food when they are not hungry just because it's there. That's good, right? And kids aren't just picky about meals; they're picky about sweets, too. There are numerous beneficial qualities of picky eaters, many of which may not be revealed until later in life.

Did you know your picky eater may make an excellent cook someday? That's because his now-sensitive taste buds can blossom into a discerning palate. In an interview on Food Republic, Michael Voltaggio, who runs one of the hottest restaurants in Los Angeles, admits to being a picky eater during childhood. When asked what he ate at age twelve, he answered, "Ramen, and grilled cheese sandwiches, and hot dogs, and chicken fingers, and the stuff that everybody else was eating. My mom actually cooked really great mom food, though. With pork chops and all that kind of stuff, she did an amazing job. I was just picky."[3]

Unfortunately, parents are repeatedly told "picky eating is bad," which creates an endless cycle. A child becomes selective. Parents panic and attempt to "get" their child to eat a certain way. The child resists. This makes picky eating even more of an issue and mealtimes more stressful, hampering the child's ability to learn and grow with food.

If this sounds familiar, you can change it. The very first step in setting yourself free from the picky-eating cycle is transforming the way you view it.

The "Picky Eating Problem" Problem

In the 1960s, two education professionals, Rosenthal and Jacobson, carried out a study in elementary school classrooms to observe the "experimenter expectancy effect."[4] Applied to the classroom, they examined how teachers' expectations affect student achievement. The kids were given an intelligence test, and 20 percent were chosen randomly. The teachers were then told this group of students had "unusual potential for intellectual growth" and were expected to do very well by the end of the year. Eight months later, they retested the students. Those that were labeled as having more potential had significantly higher test scores than the other kids not described this way.

Just viewing the average kids' potential for intelligence in a more positive light changed how the teachers treated the children. This resulted in children who did better in school compared to those viewed as less apt to learn.

Every single day this expectancy effect is in play with children and eating. When children become selective, the "picky eating" label replaces the "good eater" one. Even when children aren't told they are picky, caregivers send this message with their feeding approach: pushing, pressuring, and making special meals.

To get an idea of how this can play out, let's look at two different ways children are fed:

Scenario 1: Jake's mom thought she had a good eater until he turned three and started to refuse previously liked foods and certain meals. She feared Jake would become one of those picky kids, so she stood her ground. The food battles started – demands for more bites and using dessert as a bargaining chip – and meals gradually became the worst part of everyone's day. Different strategies were tried and failed, and there was no consistency with feeding in the home. Jake got the message that he wasn't good at eating, and he especially disliked pressure-filled family meals. Not seeing results, his mom eventually gave up, providing mostly food Jake accepted because she knew the food battles were not good for their relationship. When he reached school age, a time kids begin to open up to food, Jake stayed with his tried-and-true meals. He didn't believe he could branch out because new food had always been tied to negative experiences.

Scenario 2: Gina's mom understood picky eating was likely to show up sometime during toddlerhood, so when her two-year-old daughter started to pick at food, she didn't react at all. She kept the expectation that her daughter would eat, and family meals stayed enjoyable even on the two-bite nights. On the days Gina was done eating early, she reminded her when the next meal would be and structured her eating in a sensible way. She also knew how to boost her child's nutrition, making tweaks that helped calm her worries. She even felt inspired, as Gina would stop after eating half a bowl of ice cream, reminding her of the amazing ability of small children to regulate their food intake. By the time Gina reached school age, she started to noticeably branch out with food and felt good about eating.

You can see how each parent's outlook actually changed the atmosphere at the table, the feeding practices, and the level of confidence each child had in their eating. Unfortunately, Jake's story is much more familiar. That's because numerous articles and books tell parents picky eating is a problem that needs to be fixed. Although some strategies may work for some children, the problem is what is really behind the messages: *Parents, you can control and manipulate your child's eating.* This will almost always backfire because children can sense that they are being controlled, even if technically no one is forcing them to eat. And parents feel like failures when the strategy loses its luster or if it never works in the first place. But if the origin of picky eating is normal for most kids, then it's not a problem. The problem only occurs when we label it as a problem.

While fussy eating has always been around, its growth as a common problem is rather new. First, there is a push to get kids to eat healthy and exotic foods early. Second, parents have many different food choices, so if a child doesn't like the family dinner, it's tempting to nuke some frozen chicken nuggets as a backup. These options just weren't around in the 1950s or earlier.

Amazing things happen when you look at picky eating in a positive light and change your feeding approach. First, all that energy you put into trying to change your eater will be yours again. You can put that energy into the things you can control, like the circumstances that help children eat well (something I discuss in Chapters 3 through 7). As a result, instead of lying dormant, your child's curiosity and interest in food will begin to blossom little by little.

Once you stop viewing picky eating as a problem, you will see you have some work to do in teaching your child about food and guiding her in the right direction. Food is no different from other learned skills, like reading and writing. Kids need time, patience, and the opportunity to learn. You wouldn't expect your child to read novels at age four, so why do we expect him to eat like an adult by then?

My friends, normal picky eating is not bad, and this book will help you see it in a new, eye-opening light. But first, a little bit about me.

WHO AM I, AND WHY AM I WRITING ABOUT PICKY EATING?

As a dietitian and new mom, I had accumulated a wealth of research-based information on feeding my first child. When my second child was born in 2009, I decided to share what I had learned by starting the blog, Raise Healthy Eaters. One of my blog's first educational series was focused on picky eating. I wanted to help parents understand *why* children eat this way in the first place along with scientifically grounded strategies that help children eat better. It was well received and started a much-needed conversation.

A few years later, I ran another series focusing on what to do when picky eating doesn't get better. I found many parents struggling with kids becoming pickier over time. I also co-wrote a book entitled *Fearless Feeding: How to Raise Healthy Eaters from High Chair to High School*. I have interviewed dozens of experts, extensively reviewed research studies, and worked with families. Much of my work is grounded in international feeding expert Ellyn Satter's trust model of feeding: The Division of Responsibility (DOR).[5] While I discuss this model in Chapter 5, the idea is that children can be trusted to do their job of eating (deciding how much and whether to eat) if parents do their job of feeding (planning meals and setting the structure and locale). Feeding really can be that easy!

Perhaps nothing replaces the experience of actually being there with my own typical picky-eater kids. Strangely, I feel blessed to have middle-of-the-road eaters, meaning they are pretty average (not super picky but also not adventurous). I don't know how I could relate to parents if my kids ate everything just by my saying "take a bite." In other words: I know how you feel. My daughter, now ten years old, became pickier between two and three and started to branch out between four and five. My son, later with everything, didn't really become picky until three, and he's showing slow signs of food expansion at seven. But my kids don't know they are, or were, picky. They simply love to eat, and I have come to accept them for who they are in the eating department.

This acceptance has not always been easy. I, too, struggled with their picky ways, the ups and downs of mealtime. While I kept my cool most of the time, deep down I still felt that if I were a better cook, said the right thing at meals, or had a beautiful garden, my kids would be chowing down on broccoli.

My "aha!" moment came several years ago when a mom emailed me about her daughter, who sounded exactly the same as my girl in terms of food preferences and temperament. She did what Jake's mom did and resisted picky eating every step of the way, to the point her child was refusing to come to dinner. I realized how easily this could have been my daughter had I gone another route. Although I wanted more variety in her diet, *she was exactly where she should be.* She has grown so much since then that I'm grateful I stayed the course.

Sadly, many parents feel their kids need to eat a certain way before they can feel good about feeding them. In that case, they are going to be waiting a long time – maybe forever. Think of all that is lost during that time, including the opportunity to connect with kids and help them feel good about eating. It's not worth it to hold onto this unattainable dream that keeps us and our kids down!

This book is just as much for parents' peace of mind, as it is for helping kids. It includes information from both of my picky-eating series, the research I have gathered, and expert interviews. The book is divided into the three following sections:

THE MINDSET

The first step to viewing picky eating in a positive light is understanding why it occurs in the first place. Chapter 1 is dedicated to the current theories and research on picky eating. Chapter 2 will ease your mind because it helps you figure out if your child needs professional help for an underlying issue. Chapter 3 helps you make the very important leap from a controlling to a trusting attitude about your child's eating.

THE STRATEGIES

In Chapters 4 and 5, you'll learn the difference between the typical strategies that keep kids stuck and the empowering ones that help children learn and grow with food. Chapter 6 details how to fill nutrition gaps to help calm your worry, and help your child thrive.

THE KNOW-HOW

You're going to need help getting through the ups and downs of feeding kids. Chapter 7 showcases helpful food tips and kid-friendly recipes every parent needs in her back pocket. Chapter 8 is about giving kids hands-on experience with food, something they need, to thrive. The last two chapters, 9 and 10, include my inspirational blog posts and real-life examples of picky-to-powerful children to help you realize that your child can and will blossom where food is concerned.

LET'S BEGIN

No matter how challenging picky eating can be, I'm going to help you view it as an integral part of the feeding journey, similar to the way a child crawls before they can walk . Because, in most cases, picky eating is really just how children eat.

PART I: THE MINDSET

"The real voyage of discovery consists not of seeking new landscapes, but in having new eyes."

–Marcel Proust

Chapter 1

FROM NORMAL TO PICKY EATING

Megan had an adventurous-eating three-year-old with a hearty appetite. Over a two-month period, she noticed her daughter becoming increasingly picky; she still ate a lot, but sometimes only bread or only fruit. She even began saying, "I don't like that" to things she used to love. "I'm lucky to have read enough of your stuff to know how to handle it," she said. "But it's good for everyone to know that picky eating can happen to any child!"

Unfortunately, many parents don't understand this stage of development like Megan did, so when their child suddenly becomes more selective, it worries, disappoints, and panics them. Eating this way isn't usually problematic or something that needs to be fixed; it's a normal part of how a child develops. Instead, parents can benefit from learning to expect picky eating if they understand why it occurs in the first place.

There is no official definition of picky eating, but Kay Toomey, PhD, pediatric psychologist and developer of the

Sequential Oral Sensory (SOS) Approach to Feeding, defines it as a child who eats about 30 foods but can still tolerate new foods on his plate and eats from most food and texture groups.[1] This differentiates normal picky eaters from problem feeders who eat 20 or fewer foods and have trouble tolerating new items on their plate (discussed in Chapter 2).

THE SUPER-RESISTANT STAGE (AGE 2–6)

Here's what we know: food neophobia (fear of new food) linked with picky eating peaks between the ages of two and six.[2] In one study, 27.6 percent of three-year-olds were found to be picky eaters but this dropped to 13.6 percent at six years.[3] That doesn't mean picky eating disappears by age six, but it generally gets better as kids enter school. During the picky stage, children drop some of the foods they used to eat and become resistant to anything they view as new or different.

One way to truly grasp what is going on is to look at eating from the perspective of your child, along with the supporting research:

The Erratic Eater: *I know everyone wants me to eat, but I'm just not that hungry. As a baby, I wanted food all the time, but now that I'm a toddler, I'm just not into eating as much.*

The Facts: After one year, the rapid growth that occurred in infancy will start to slow down. Birth weight triples in the first year of life but then doesn't quadruple until the second year. Children between age two and puberty gain an average of 4.5–6.5 pounds per year. This change shows up in their meal patterns, which can include days in which they seem disinterested in food. As long as their growth is on track, you can't expect your child to eat the same amounts at each meal.[4]

The Afraid-to-Eat Kid: *New foods and certain textures scare me. I'm afraid that something bad will happen if I eat it. I wish my parents wouldn't push it so much. Maybe watching them eat these foods a bunch of times will help me calm down.*

The Facts: "The thinking is that food neophobia has evolved to protect kids as they become more mobile and are able to ingest foods," said Jennifer Orelet Fisher, PhD, Associate Professor at the Department of Public Health at Temple University. Fisher explained how this developmental phase may have been adapted from a time when fear of strange foods kept kids from eating harmful toxins. Even though people no longer hunt for food, kids are biologically driven to be skeptical of unfamiliar foods. She said food neophobia will vary in children and often matches temperament, so you might see a cautious kid also cautious about new foods and a more easy-going one less afraid.

The Strong-Willed Child: *I know my parents did everything for me when I was younger, but I'm older now and want some say in the matter. Plus, food seems to be such a hot-button issue!*

The Facts: Picky eating typically starts in toddlerhood, when kids are beginning to understand they are a separate person from their parents. They will test their limits during mealtime as they establish a sense of autonomy. This is a normal part of development.

The Veggie Resister: *I know my mom wants me to eat broccoli and other green vegetables, but the bitter taste is too much for me to take.*

The Facts: "We all experience different taste worlds," said Alexandra Logue, PhD, Research Professor in The Center for the Advanced Study of Education (CASE) at the Graduate Center of The City University of New York and author of *The Psychology of Eating and Drinking.* "There's a strong genetic component to taste preferences. It's not kids' or parents' fault." Logue is referring to supertasters, who naturally taste lower concentrations of certain chemicals, making them sensitive to the taste and texture of particular foods. She has firsthand experience; by age one, she would only eat bread and milk.

"I can remember as a kid how intense the flavors were," she said. Now as an adult, Logue will eat anything except fish. Research shows that 70 percent of preschoolers are sensitive to the bitter compounds found in many vegetables called 6-n-propothiouricil (PROP), which is why young children often shun vegetables (strategies on how to combat this in Chapters 6 and 7).[5] One study showed both genetic and environmental effects on food preferences but found liking fruit, vegetables, and proteins is more likely to be genetically linked, while preferences for starchy foods, snack foods, and dairy are more likely to be due to a child's food environment.[6]

The Carb Lover: *There are some foods that are just easier to like and fill me up with less effort.*

The Facts: "Children have evolved to like sweet foods," said Fisher. "That's why fruits are highly acceptable and easy to like, while vegetables are the least preferred." Fisher said children are actually hardwired to prefer sweet and energy-rich foods. To kids, sweetness signals a food is calorie dense, while sour and bitter tastes indicate it might be harmful. Although this is true, kids (and adults) can learn to like vegetables through exposure and positive experiences.

The Growing Child: *It's weird, but there are times I just could eat and eat. I get the feeling my parents want me to always eat the same amount, but sometimes my body is telling me it needs more.*

The Facts: While growth rates slow after the first year of life, kids will periodically go through growth spurts where they eat more than they usually do. The two biggest spurts of growth occur during infancy and puberty, but all kids go through periods when they are growing faster and other times when they aren't. Appetite is linked to growth. As long as your child's growth is steady, don't let changes in appetite alarm you.

The "I'm Not Ready" Child: *I love my parents. They are super cool. I want to eat like them, but I'm just not ready. Someday I'll get there.*

The Facts: In her book *Child of Mine: Feeding with Love and Good Sense*, Ellyn Satter writes how kids really do want to eat like their parents, even when it seems otherwise:

Because he thinks that you are great and have all the answers, when he sees you eating green beans, he reasons that eating green beans must be the thing to do. You don't have to say another word. All you have to do is enjoy your green beans. Observing that, your child will assume that someday he, too, will eat green beans.[7]

The Inexperienced Eater: *I cringe when I see meat on my plate. I know I have all my teeth and have been chewing for awhile, but I still prefer my meats moist and cut up some of the time.*

The Facts: By the time kids reach preschool age, parents may assume they can chew and swallow like adults, but these skills aren't fully mastered until later in childhood. Children can more easily lose track of food in their mouth, are still developing mastication (chewing) and their airway is smaller than adults.[8] Tough meats and round foods like hot dogs are especially problematic.

The bottom-line is that your child is acting this way around food because he is changing both physically and mentally, not because he is trying to be a pain or because of something you did.

KNOW WHAT TO EXPECT AT EACH STAGE OF DEVELOPMENT

Up until now, we have focused on the time picky eating usually starts, but it's important to have a big-picture view of what to expect at each stage of development. This helps the mom of a three-year-old know that her child will expand his eating with time and exposure. It also helps a parent of an older child look back to see where problems occurred. Here is a summary of what you can expect in terms of normal development:

Infancy (0–2 years): In *Fearless Feeding*, my coauthor and I call this the honeymoon phase of eating.[9] Most babies (but not all) are open to a variety of foods and textures. They also have big appetites and show up ready to eat. This is a good time to get a variety of food in front of your child.

Toddler & Preschooler (2–5 years): During the super-resistant stage, growth slows and minds develop, causing children to not only eat erratically but to be skeptical of unfamiliar foods. They may even drop some previously liked foods. Kids are also becoming more sensitive to environmental cues of eating (asking for sweets, etc.).

School Age (6–12 years): During this stage, children gradually expand their food choices, but they are also influenced by friends. Growth is stable until puberty starts (age 10–11 for girls and 11–12 for boys) when appetite and growth accelerate.

Teenager (13–18 years): Adolescents open up even more with food, but they also want to be different and may try trendy diets like being vegetarian or even weight loss (be careful). Growth and appetite continue to climb.

If your child seems out of the norm, there are a few things to consider. First, a baby who had trouble accepting food from the beginning may have something else going on, either physically or sensory-wise. The older child still eating few foods may have underlying issues, too (see Chapter 2).

Although the school-age child who isn't expanding his food intake may just be a late bloomer, it also could be the way he has been fed since becoming picky, increasing the shelf life of fussy eating. Chapter 5 includes a discussion of the feeding approaches that backfire, like pressuring to eat, that could be at the root of the issue.

What typically occurs during the school years is children gradually open up to food. Yes, their peers may influence them, but their appetite and mind grows. They slowly outgrow food neophobia as they gain more experiences with food. One positive experience builds on the next. For example, you might see your child trying more food without eating more than a bite or two, but over time, that one bite turns into three, which leads to eventual acceptance.

A WORD ON CHILD DIFFERENCES

The simple fact that all kids are different is something missing from messages about picky eating. While parents have a strong influence over their child's eating over time, each child comes into the world with his own unique way of relating to food. Figuring out what that is, and working around it, can help parents and children immensely.

In *Fearless Feeding,* my coauthor and I showcase three different types of eating styles that are most likely to occur in children. The first is the eager eater, the child who generally accepts a wide variety of food. This child often has a big appetite and may not go through much of a picky-eating phase. Then there is the extra-cautious eater. This child often has a low appetite and is very careful around food, which may have started when solids were introduced. These children may be "super tasters" who are much more sensitive to the taste and texture of foods. Most kids (including mine) fall somewhere in between these two eating styles. These kids eat a lot the first two years of life then may become resistant, as previously mentioned, but gradually expand their food intake. I call them "by the book" eaters.

Family history contributes to the kind of eater you have, as research shows that fear of new food is highly genetically linked.[10] So if you or your partner were picky as a child, for example, it is likely your child will be, too. "Pickiness seems to be shockingly genetic, according to what I've seen. Almost without exception, the picky eaters I hear about have at least one parent who was very picky as well," said Sheila Kelly, MS, RD, of SkellySkills.com. "A lot of times they don't realize this until I ask them. Then, when they remember how picky they were, and realize that they eat a decent diet now, they seem to not worry as much about it."

There's also the issue of temperament, which is why some easygoing children do well with a one-bite or taste rule and other (more stubborn) kids don't. What I have found is that the pickier kids tend to respond less well to pressure of any sort (discussed in Chapter 5). That's why advice like, "Just have him take one bite" doesn't work for everyone and can often backfire on the very kids who need help.

As a parent, you already know your child's eating style extremely well. If you find yourself constantly frustrated, it's probably because you are attempting to change an eating personality that is unchangeable. Maybe you are trying hard to get your cautious eater to be an eager eater, pushing your stubborn child to try new foods, or trying to make your "loves-to-eat" child eat smaller amounts like other kids.

The good news is that all kids can grow up to be healthy and happy eaters, but the road to get there will be different for each unique child. This book will provide you with the tools you need to be successful.

HOW KIDS EAT

The goal of this chapter is to shift your thinking from "picky eating is a problem" to "picky eating is how most kids eat." Whether your child is middle of the road or extra cautious, you now have a realistic base from which to draw. But there is a minority of kids whose picky eating is due to

Chapter 2

FROM DOUBT TO PEACE OF MIND

Lindsay was enjoying parenthood like any mom when she noticed something about the way her child accepted food. "I started suspecting that my son (now three years old) was having atypical difficulties with feeding when he was between twelve and fifteen months of age," she said. "He would eat any type of smoothly puréed foods as a baby, but then really struggled with textured purées. He really wouldn't tolerate much of anything and would spit out everything we tried giving him."

Lindsay Lapaquette, Speech-Language Pathologist (SLP) and Director of the West Island Speech Clinic, had her son diagnosed with sensory processing disorder at 21 months of age and a daughter diagnosed at seven months. She asked the question almost every parent of a picky eater asks at one time or another: *Is my child's picky eating normal or not?* That is the question I want to help you answer.

10 RED FLAGS EVERY PARENT SHOULD KNOW

There are different terms used to describe a child who is unusually picky; the most common terms are problem feeder, resistant eater, and selective eater. Kay Toomey, PhD, introduced in Chapter 1, defines problem feeders as children who consume 20 or fewer foods and will reject whole texture categories.[1] A problem feeder might yell and scream when near disliked foods, won't graduate to new textures, and may gag or vomit after eating certain foods. Below is a list of common red flags. [2] If your child exhibits one or more of these signs, it could indicate a problem.

1. Poor weight gain, falling percentages on growth chart
2. Coughing, gagging, or choking during meals
3. Problems with vomiting
4. Unable to take puréed food by ten months
5. Unable to take finger foods by one year
6. Not drinking from a cup by sixteen months
7. Accepting fewer than 20 foods
8. Avoiding foods in one texture or food group
9. Crying at most meals (for infants) or having tantrums about new foods (for older children)
10. Frequent family fights about food

(For a full list, see http://www.sosapproach-conferences.comarticles/red-flags.)

"Meals were extremely stressful in our household," said Lapaquette. "My son would start tantruming before dinner had even begun, screaming that he wanted a preferred food rather than what was being served."

The American Psychiatric Association changed the diagnostic criteria for problematic picky eating from "feeding disorder of infancy or early childhood" to "avoidant/restrictive food intake disorder" (ARFID) in their Diagnostic and Statistical Manual of Mental Disorders (DSM-5).[3] The change was made because this disorder is not just for young children; it can occur after age six and into adulthood. ARFID should not be confused with eating disorders like bulimia nervosa or anorexia nervosa because weight and shape are not driving forces behind food refusal.

"While his twin sister would pick mushrooms, peppers, and different meats off my plate, my son showed no interest in food or eating. He never complained of hunger. Ever," said Skye van Zetten, who blogs at Mealtime Hostage. "When we insisted he try some of our meal, he would cry and hide behind his chair. Our doctor said he would grow out of it."

Resistant eaters aren't trying to be difficult, they are trying to let their parents know that eating hurts or is difficult for them.

UNDERSTANDING THE WHY

Once the signs are identified, it's important to discover the why behind the child's avoidance of eating. In Lapaquette's case, her kids had sensory processing disorder, which is difficulty processing the sensory properties of food's smell, taste, and texture. Van Zetten's son had several choking incidents that seemed to be a contributing factor, and he dropped acceptance of foods after each incident.

"Problematic picky eating is commonly caused by an undiagnosed gastrointestinal issue (reflux, constipation, allergies), an undiagnosed oral/motor disorder (muscle weakness or coordination issues for chewing), or a sensory processing disorder," said Jennifer Hatfield, an SLP who works with resistant eaters. "While less common, it can be triggered by well-meaning caregivers who have taken bad advice for their very cautious eater (force them to try something new, only serve 'healthy' foods and they'll eat them, or refuse to give in and they'll eventually eat)."

If it's a medical issue or a reaction to a past incident, like reflux or choking, the child still may be very cautious around food even when the condition is controlled. Children with autism spectrum disorder, ADHD, or developmental delays are much more likely to experience difficulty eating. While the causes may be different, the key behind every resistant eater is an intense, very real fear of eating food.

WHAT ABOUT OLDER PICKY EATERS?

"Older picky eaters are no different than younger picky eaters when it comes to reasons. The difference is that it affects them more socially because of how food-oriented our 'social' time is," said Hatfield. "Think about a teen who gets invited to a party but is an extremely picky eater. How do you navigate all of those foods you don't like as well as the questions from others as to why you aren't eating? You'll look 'different,' and that is devastating to an adolescent. Same for adults."

Diane Keddy, MS, RD, FAED works with selective eaters of all ages, but quite a few that are older, like age ten. The reason kids get treatment late is that growth may be steady, so pediatricians tell parents to wait it out. "Most pediatricians are missing it," said Keddy. "The longer parents wait to get help, the harder it is to treat." Keddy describes these kids as only accepting a very narrow range of (usually white) food. The typical list includes pasta, macaroni and cheese, goldfish crackers, and milk.

Another red flag: selective eaters tend to only eat their accepted foods at home, even if someone else is making it the exact same way. When they try a new food, it's common for them to choke, gag, or even vomit, which leads to anxiety about eating. Keddy explains that this reaction is neurological because the part of their brain that recognizes food as pleasure is underdeveloped.

"Children with a family history of autism, eating disorders, obsessive compulsive disorder, and severe picky eating are at greater risk for developing selective eating," she said. "With autism spectrum disorders on the rise, selective eating is becoming more common."

GETTING THE RIGHT HELP

For her son and daughter, Lapaquette chose SOS feeding therapy she describes as having a "significant impact" on meals in her house. The idea is getting children comfortable with food by gradually introducing and exposing them in non-stressful ways.

Van Zetten had a different experience. After visiting two dietitians and working with occupational therapists, a bad flu caused her son to dip below the 5th percentile for weight; she stopped therapy and embraced the trust model of feeding by following Ellyn Satter's Division of Responsibility. Her son's diet increased from 13 to 27 unique foods, and his weight is now at the 18th percentile.

In her practice, Diane Keddy utilizes a treatment called "systematic desensitization" that is very different than what she recommends for normal picky-eating kids. She describes it as a negotiation where kids are allowed so many "pass" foods. She says the treatment takes a lot of energy and commitment from parents, but it's worth it because many kids do well.

This shows that different treatments work for different kids. In their book, *Helping Your Child with Extreme Picky Eating,* Dr. Katja Rowell and speech therapist Jenny McGlothlin, write that while therapy is helpful in the right circumstances, if children resist or are pushed beyond their comfort level, it can worsen picky eating and decrease appetite. Rowell and McGlothlin help parents recognize when therapy is not helping: "If it increases anxiety, gagging, vomiting, or power struggles, or you are negotiating every agonizing bite, that's counterproductive." They recommend opening a dialogue with prospective feeding therapy partners by asking key questions:

- What is their training?
- What type of approach do they use?
- How long have they been working with feeding?
- Are they aware of the Division of Responsibility, The Get Permission Approach or Responsive Feeding?
- What is considered "successful" treatment? What criteria determine when treatment is over?
- What can therapists offer if a child resists?
- What support is offered to parents at home?

Help can come from a pediatric dietitian, a dietitian specializing in eating disorders, a speech pathologist (SLP), an occupation therapist (OT), or a feeding team that includes various members (dietitian, OT/SLP, and psychologist). "If a parent has pursued intervention and has not yet had success, maybe they didn't have the right therapist, or maybe they only got a piece of the answer from the therapist they saw," said Lapaquette.

I wish the answer was simple and that there was one therapy that works with every resistant eater out there. The key is to find out if you have a resistant eater in the first place, why the problem is occurring, and trust your gut when it comes to finding help.

This book is written for typical picky eaters that do not have underlying issues affecting their eating. That doesn't mean it can't be helpful for a child in feeding therapy, but it shouldn't replace advice from a healthcare provider. Below are resources that can help.

PARENT SUPPORT
Mealtime Hostage has a closed parent-to-parent Facebook support group for parents of selective eating children who are learning about and getting started with Division Of Responsibility feeding.
https://www.facebook.com/groups/MealtimeHostage

FINDING HELP
- Food for Thought blog
  http://foodforthoughtlinds.blogspot.com/
- Find an SLP or OT who specializes in feeding (may be listed as dysphagia) http://www.asha.org/findpro/
- Find a dietitian
  http://www.eatright.org/iframe/findrd.aspx
- Find an SOS therapist http://www.sosapproach-conferences.com/parents/find-an-sos-therapist
- Melanie Potock's My Munch Bug
  http://www.mymunchbug.com/
- Jennifer Hatfield's Therapy and Learning Services
  https://www.therapyandlearningservices.com/
- West Island Speech http://www.westislandspeech.ca/
- Marsha Dunn Klein at Mealtime Notions
  http://mealtimenotions.com/about/

BOOKS
- *Helping Your Child with Extreme Picky Eating: A*

Step-by-Step Guide for Overcoming Selective Eating, Food Aversion and Feeding Disorders by Katja Rowell and Jennifer McGlothlin

- *Fearless Feeding: How to Raise Healthy Eaters from High Chair to High School* (Chapter 7) by Jill Castle and Maryann Jacobsen
- *Love Me, Feed Me: The Adoptive Parents Guide to Ending the Worry About Weight, Picky Eating, Power Struggles and More* (Chapters 3 & 4) by Katja Rowell
- *Raising a Happy and Healthy Eater: A Stage-by-Stage Guide to Setting Your Child on the Path to Adventurous Eating* by Nimali Fernando and Melanie Potock
- *Food Chaining: The Proven 6-Step Plan to Stop Picky Eating, Solve Feeding Problems, and Expand Your Child's Diet* by Cheryl Fraker, Mark Fishbein, Sibyl Cox and Laura Walbert
- *Just Take a Bite: Easy, Effective Answers to Food Aversions and Eating Challenges* by Lori Emsperger, Tania Stegen-Hanson, and Temple Grandin

PEACE OF MIND

The goal of this chapter is to give you peace of mind and tools to determine if your child needs help or not. If you have doubts, get an evaluation. If you don't, let's move on to Chapter 3!

Chapter 3

FROM CONTROLLING TO TRUSTING ATTITUDE

J ennifer realized her attitude about picky eating had a direct effect on the atmosphere at her family's table. "One of the feeding issues I had was with me. I realized that I was the one that was panicking when I made a meal and he wouldn't even try it," she said. "I would be so worried he wasn't getting enough nutrients. Once I let that go, and let him set the pace of trying new foods, our meals became so much less stressful."

When you see picky eating as a problem, like Jennifer did, you are more likely to try to control or cater to kids out of fear. When you view picky eating as a normal part of growing up, and also as part of a child's unique eating personality, the dynamic changes completely.

One way to think about feeding your child is to consider the components needed to grow a plant. To be successful, you need the right kind of soil, seeds, light, and water. If just one of these items is missing, the plant doesn't bloom right, and in some cases, it may not grow at all. But all plants are different; some bloom sooner or much later than others. Your overall attitude toward your child's eating is like soil for a plant. You want the most nutrient-rich soil from which all growth stems. In feeding, this nutrient-rich soil is trust and acceptance.

TRUST AND ACCEPTANCE LAY THE FOUNDATION

Let's say a good friend tells you her most precious secret while stressing how much she trusts you. Doesn't that make you want to live up to her expectations, guarding the secret extra tight? That's how trust works. When we trust our kids to move along food acceptance at their own pace, we send the message that they can do it. When we distrust them – push, prod, or make things too easy – we send the opposite message.

Trust = You can do it!
Distrust = You can't do it!

Parents generally trust that their children will eventually do lots of things like walk, talk, read and write, but when it comes to food, this trust gets challenging. It's simply harder for parents to believe their child will eat well without some interference on their part. Kids can eat well and enjoy healthy food, but trust is an integral part of the process.

Unconditional acceptance goes hand in hand with trust because when a picky eater feels his being accepted is contingent on his eating, it can negatively impact his feelings of self-worth and his relationship with you. Coming to the table is no longer about getting nourished, it's about feeling accepted by the most important people in his life, and that sure is a lot of pressure.

"I grew up as an extremely picky eater. I didn't like being picky; it made a lot of social situations very difficult," said Kia Robertson, creator of Today I Ate a Rainbow, an educational kit that gets kids excited about healthy eating. "I'm sure it would be very challenging for a parent that has never been picky to 'deal' with a picky eater, but when you can take a compassionate approach and see eating from a child's point of view, I think it helps to give parents more patience and understanding."

There's also an upside to accepting your child's "no," according to a 2004 piece in *The Permanente Journal*:

...By accepting their children's refusal to eat a particular food at a particular time or their lack of a big appetite at a particular meal, parents send the message not only that using No is okay in this family but also that you can use No and still be loved in this family. This method of parenting is powerful because it builds within children a deeper sense of connection with their parents as well as internal beliefs that differ from those of children whose No is ignored or overridden. A child whose parents accept No will later be much more likely to feel comfortable saying No to something that is not good for the child.[1]

The typical food battles that result from trying to change a child take the joy and connection out of eating. Some parents may win the battle and feel good that their child eats the way they want him to eat, but deep down, the child may be full of resentment, eating peas to please his parents and not because he enjoys eating them.

The first step in helping your child is choosing trust, acceptance, and understanding over control and fear. This isn't about giving up. It's about creating a supportive environment that maximizes a child's ability to learn and grow with food.

Watch Those Labels

At the grocery store, I saw a young girl pick up raspberries asking her mom to buy them. "Why do you want these? You NEVER eat raspberries when I buy them," the mom replied in a stern tone. What the mom didn't understand was that this is how children learn to like different foods. They see it several times, they show interest, they don't eat if for a while, they try a bite, they don't eat it for a while, they try it again, and so on. This mom was telling her daughter she didn't like raspberries, but that wasn't true. Her daughter was going through the process of food learning, the same way kids learn to do other things like read and write. This is a good example of the Expectancy Effect we talked about in the introduction. The "picky" label changes how children view their own ability to eat well.

Instead of using labels like "picky," we can remind children (and ourselves) that they are learning about food and not react at all to their food choices. "The constant reminders not to pressure and that picky eating is one stage of normal development have really helped," said Katie. "My daughter even told the doctor at her well check to check her taste buds and see how much they've grown! That's how we frame it at home when she doesn't care for something the rest of us like, that her taste buds are still growing like the rest of her and will get there."

It can be tough to keep offering food you know your child is unlikely to eat, but by doing so, you not only expose him to food (an important part of learning), you help instill confidence. "If mom and dad believe in me, maybe I can do it."

Instead of "you probably won't like this," or "you are so picky," always serve food with an expectant attitude and avoid making comments about your child's eating. This high-expectancy attitude (minus the judgment) will positively affect your child's relationship with food.

ENJOYMENT VERSUS EATING PERFORMANCE

In *Fearless Feeding,* my coauthor and I estimate that parents will feed their children about 28,000 times before they reach adulthood and leave the house.[2] As kids get older, mealtime may be the only time parents get to connect with their children. If these meals are tense or all about how or what a child eats, an important connection gets lost. Instead of focusing on what your child is eating, take the time to enjoy quality time with her. Don't forget: your job is done once you place the meal on the table.

"You've prepared a delicious and considerate meal for your family. Once you serve it, your time to worry about the food is over," wrote Skye van Zetten on her blog Mealtime Hostage. "Sit down and enjoy the company at the table. If you are like most modern families, dinner is the first chance you've had to talk to each other."

When meals are enjoyable, it bolsters the feeding relationship defined by Ellyn Satter as *"the complex interactions that takes place between parent and child as they engage in food selection, ingestion, and regulation behaviors."*[3] Strengthening the feeding relationship will help improve the overall relationship with your child, inadvertently helping him develop his eating habits.

Another way to keep meals pleasant is to focus less on the behaviors you don't want and more on the ones you do. When little Kate says how "gross" a food is, remind her to simply say, "No, thank you." If a child refuses to eat, that's fine, but let him know he needs to come to the table for a period of time. Just don't engage in the "you-have-to-eat" battle.

The best soil for your child to bloom with food is infused with trust, high expectations, and joyful meals. You may not be able to hear it, but your child will be thinking, "Eating and cooking are fun," "Mom and Dad accept me for who I am, so I can eat new food when I'm ready," and "They believe I can do it, so I believe I can do it."

THE TRUST MINDSET

This is pretty powerful stuff. Now that you have the mindset down, it's time move into the specific research-based strategies that will help your child learn and grow with food.

PART II: THE STRATEGIES

"Strategy is just a fancy for word for coming up with a long-term plan and putting it into action."

– Ellie Pedot

Chapter 4

FROM CHAOTIC TO CONSISTENT OFFERINGS

Mandi knew her seven-year-old son didn't care for chicken. But since the rest of her family liked it, she served it every so often along with other foods. "Last night my son asked if he could eat his with ketchup, even though I didn't serve it that way. Yes, absolutely," she said. "Even though I had other things on the table that he enjoys and figured he'd probably skip the chicken, he ended up eating a decent portion of it."

Food acceptance happens when food is offered repeatedly without pressure. It may not happen overnight, but it occurs often when parents least expect it. Mandi was surprised, but she really shouldn't be—she had been creating the circumstances to help her child grow with food for some time.

Now that you have the right soil, you need to plant the seeds. Not just any seeds; they need to be the right kind, so your child will bloom to her potential. You can't make your child eat, but you can create the circumstances that allow her to eat well, which includes meal structure, selecting and storing food, and serving meals.

STRUCTURING MEALS AND SNACKS

The first key component is structure, a regular and consistent offering of food. Having routine meals and snacks in a designated area, instead of grazing or giving in to food requests, helps children regulate their food intake, ask for food less often, and feel secure about eating. According to one study, the more children accumulated eating behaviors that weren't structured, like skipping breakfast, snacking between meals, and watching TV while eating, the higher their weights were.[1]

Feeding babies on demand makes sense, but it doesn't work for older children. Toddlers don't always know how to communicate hunger until they melt down, and older kids can use pretend hunger to get what they want (my son used to say he was hungry for chocolate). Additionally, this type of feeding can also lead to grazing and poor behavior at mealtime.

How often should kids eat? By one year, most children are eating about six times per day, with the last meal typically consisting of milk or a breastfeeding session. Toddlers tend to eat every two-to-three hours (five-to-six meals per day), while preschoolers may be able to go three or even four hours between meals. Sample meal plans, like those in the American Academy of Pediatrics *Pediatric Nutrition Handbook*, recommend three main meals and two between-meal snacks for the average toddler or preschooler.[2]

By school age, children can move to three meals and one afternoon snack, but timing of breakfast and lunch matter. For example, a child that starts school early (7:30 a.m., meaning breakfast is at seven or earlier) but doesn't have lunch until 12:30 p.m. would need to eat something in between. Of course, each child is different, so individualizing is important.

Toddler: 5–6 times per day (3 meals and 2–3 snacks)
Preschooler: 5 times per day (3 meals and 2 snacks)
School Age: 4–5 times per day (3 meals and 1–2 snacks)

Structuring meals and snacks without eating in between helps kids come to the table with an appetite. It also helps them get the right amount of food for their body type and decreases the likelihood they will eat for reasons other than hunger, such as boredom or upset feelings.

GET FAMILY MEALS GOING

Family meals combine the benefits of repeated exposure with role modeling. It also teaches kids how to behave at the dinner table and gives families time to connect. I know your schedules may be wacky, but get this habit going as soon as you can.

Kathleen Cuneo, PhD, says that switching from special kid meals to family meals was the turning point for her now-teenage daughter. "I saw a positive change when I stopped nagging her and we made a commitment to family meals," she said."When I backed off and she was expected to eat from what was made available, she became open to trying new foods."

Family dinners may not automatically change your child's eating, but research supports the benefits, from lowering the risk of eating disorders to healthier eating.[3] Try to eat together when you can: lunches and breakfasts work, too. Serving meals in a way everyone can enjoy is key to everyone's sanity, and it's discussed in the following section.

FAMILY-FRIENDLY FEEDING

Lisa Gross, dietitian and mom of three, said that when her daughter was two and turned ultra picky, she was tempted to provide her with only her favorites (she loved pasta!). "I just kept offering the same food we ate but always offered fruit, bread, and some accompaniment that she would eat," she said. "I hoped that she would outgrow this stage, and now that she's five, it's much better."

We've discussed how truly scared kids can be in trying new foods. So, while you don't want kids to dictate the menu, you also want them to look down at their plate and see something that is familiar. When planning the menu, consider the whole family. Sometimes dinner may be a kid's favorite, and other nights it will be a parent's favorite. Try to have at least one or two items at the table that your child is likely to eat on nights when the main course is not his favorite. A good night to try different sides is when he likes the main dish.

Family-style meals also help: serve items separately in bowls and allow children to serve themselves (with help from parents as needed). In addition to giving kids the control they crave, family-style meals help those younger than six who have a need for things to be "just right" and prefer foods that don't touch.

Once you get into a routine, you can build on foods and flavors children already accept. If a child likes breaded items, for example, try breading zucchini or fish with the same spices (this is how my daughter learned to like fish; I made them fish nuggets!). Got a kid who likes burritos with meat? Consider making the same dish with chicken or shrimp. Make small changes instead of big ones and be patient. Research suggests that children are more likely to accept new foods if they are similar to other recipes and flavors they enjoy.[4] Below are my top tips for family-friendly meals.

- *Serve family-style meals:* Place bowls of food on the table and pass around. Your child will feel empowered serving himself!
- *Choose theme nights with predictable sides:* Plan Mexican, Italian, fish, soup, and grill nights (some are seasonal). Always include sides kids accept, such as tortillas and beans on Mexican night and bread and meatballs on Italian night.
- *Check in with kids on meal prep:* When making modifiable items like quesadillas, check in with your child about ingredients. If he doesn't want tomatoes, skip them in the quesadilla but still serve them on the side.
- *Modify salads and veggies:* Does your child dislike vinaigrette dressing? Serve her salad (naked) with a side of ranch or let her make her own salad. Serve raw veggies next to cooked ones with yummy sauces for dipping.
- *Build flavors and meals kids like:* Look for new meals that include a sauce or well-liked food to help bridge the gap to the new food, such as breaded items or a favorite pasta sauce.
- *Teach kids what to say:* Let kids know it's not acceptable to say food is "yucky" or "gross." A simple "No, thank you" will do.

Due to their developmental need to have things "just right," many young children don't prefer mixed dishes like casseroles. That doesn't mean you don't serve them, but consider separating ingredients out if possible (sauce on the side) or encouraging your child to pick out the foods they like, such as the lasagna noodles. This gradually exposes them to the dish, and over time, they are likely to eat more.

When Alexandra (now an adult) first started eating salad as a child, her mom put a lot of her favorite dressing in a bowl with a small amount of vegetables. Over time, the dressing quantity decreased and the vegetables increased. That is how she learned to like salads.

Instead of plopping a foreign meal down and expecting your child to eat it, make it a habit to have something he can eat and be strategic about expanding his food base. Your powerful little eater will appreciate it!

A Word on Catering and Variety

Board-certified pediatric dietitian Angela Lemond, RD, explains that the most common feeding mistake she sees in her practice is short-order cooking: making another meal when children say they don't like what's being served. "Parents are so concerned kids won't get the nutrition they need that they operate out of fear," she said. "They don't realize that letting their kids decide what to eat exacerbates the issue."

In the book *Child of Mine*, Ellyn Satter explains it this way:

Making an alternative food so readily available tells your child louder than words can say, "I don't expect you to learn to eat your meals." Remember that your child wants to grow up with respect to eating, but she will take the easy way out if it is offered.[5]

What about variety? A good rule of thumb is to try and not serve the same meal two days in a row. If yesterday was peanut butter and jelly for lunch, today can be a turkey sandwich. "I found this a bit tough, particularly in the beginning when they ate so few foods, so I just tried my best to keep food repetition as minimal as possible over two days," says Lindsay Lapaquette, introduced in Chapter 2. "But even now, with them having a bigger repertoire, I see the impact."

Just as a plant cannot grow without seeds, a child cannot grow without regular food offerings, a variety of food from which to choose, and watching more experienced eaters eat. But even when parents do this well, they can get into trouble by pushing their child to eat. Let's take a look at this in the next chapter.

Chapter 5

FROM PICKY TO POWERFUL
FEEDING APPROACH

Jane realized the pressure she had put on her nine-year-old son all these years wasn't working. She required him to eat at least half of his favorites, like chicken, and she would have him eat a certain number of bites in order to have dessert. She also required tastes of food, and while she tried her best to make meals pleasant, they were often tense. This pressure got him to eat the required amount at meals, but he wasn't branching out on his own, and his weight remained low.

Like a lot of parents, Jane tried to speed up the process of food acceptance. But by doing so, her son never moved forward. This is very typical of picky children and this chapter will dig into *why*.

You've got your soil (attitude) and your seeds (food structure and offerings), and now it's time to allow for the right amount of water and sunlight (feeding approach). Every plant is different; some need more water and sun while others require much less. If you pour too much water

on the wrong type of plant, it will not grow right. You have
fed it today, but you've kept it from eventually blooming.

THE DIVISION OF RESPONSIBILITY GIVES YOUR CHILD ROOM TO GROW

While some kids do okay with pushes, pickier kids typically
don't because they are more sensitive to the taste and
texture of food, and may need more time to feel
comfortable. In one study, children who were less picky
were more likely to accept a novel fruit with modeling and
prompting. Yet the pickier children did best with the
modeling only (no prompting).[1] They are like plants that
need extra time to grow without too much food or sunlight.

A quick word about motivation: most kids are not
motivated to eat just by being told to do so. When you leave
the choice up to children, they decide to eat because they
want to, and that is very internally motivating. This is why
Satter's Division of Responsibility (DOR) works so well; it
gives children reasonable freedom and choice.[2] Although
kids don't get to choose the meal, they do get to choose
whether or not to eat and how much to eat from what is
served. Most feeding problems occur when parent or child
crosses the Division of Responsibility.

Satter's Division of Responsibility	
Parent's Job	*Child's Job*
• Decide what to serve while considering child's food preferences	• Decide what to eat from what is served at meal or snack time
• Decide when the family eats and where, such as at the kitchen table	• Decide how much to eat based on feelings of hunger and fullness

Even though DOR is supported by the American Academy of Pediatrics and other major health organizations, it's not used frequently. In fact, according to one study, 85 percent of parents try to get their children to eat more using rewards and praise.[3] In other words, the pressure to eat is a frequent guest at many dinner tables across America. At the family table, the aim is to get a child to eat something or eat in a way that a caregiver deems acceptable.

Parents will often say, "I don't make my kids eat," but they forget about the negative effects of pressure, both covert and overt. For example, covert pressure might be having a child cook or help in the garden with the sole intention of getting them to eat (offering tastes of food at every corner). Overt pressure might be saying something like, "Come on, eat it, I worked hard on this meal." Pressure can take many forms, but what really matters isn't what the parents say but how the child receives it.

Studies show that children who are slow to eat and underweight are the most likely to be pressured to eat.[4] And guess what? That pressure produces the opposite of what parents want: a loss of appetite. Because picky children are more sensitive to the taste and texture of food, just the thought of everyone staring at them, trying to get them to eat, makes eating less appetizing. "The main thing to remember with a reluctant eater is that much of their issues with food are due to anxiety, which can trigger the fight or flight response, decreasing appetite," said Jennifer Hatfield, SLP, introduced in Chapter 2. "Pressure not only causes a behavioral response, but it also causes an actual chemical change in how the body flips the switch *off* on the very thing we are trying desperately to switch *on*."

Take a study published in *Appetite*. Children pressured to eat soup not only ate less, they made 157 negative comments while eating compared to 30 negative comments in the no-pressure group, coloring the eating atmosphere as negative.[5]

Parents can choose encouragement instead of pressure. This is showing kids you believe in them and providing helpful ideas while making it clear that the choice to eat is ultimately theirs. Examples of encouragement versus pressure are listed below:

Encouragement: "These potatoes are kind of like that other potato dish you like. I think you'll like them."
Pressure: "They are just potatoes...try them!"

Encouragement: "This looks really tasty. Here you go."
Pressure: "You'll disappoint the cook if you don't eat at least some of this meal."

Encouragement: "If you aren't ready to take a bite of the soup, you can take out the noodle pieces with your hands."
Pressure: "It has chicken and noodles: how can you not want to eat that??"

Encouragement: "Remember, if you decide to take a bite and don't like it, you can carefully spit it out in your napkin, or you can try licking or touching it first."
Pressure: "You can't leave the table until you take a bite."

Checking back a few months later, Jane, introduced at the beginning of the chapter, admits that "it takes patience and diligence," but she's leaving it up to her son to decide what and how much of what she serves to eat at mealtime. He's added a couple of foods to his 'likes' list, including sweet potatoes and grapes, and he is also drinking more milk. It's slow progress but it's progress made by a willing child, and that's the difference.

It Takes More Than You Think to Work Up to That Bite

The one-bite rule is one piece of advice you've probably heard again and again: *just make them take a bite or taste.* Some less-picky children may view a one-bite rule as the push they need to try new things, while others will be totally put off by it. If just having kids taste food worked for every kid, there would be no picky kids out there.

"In my experience as a feeding specialist, the one-bite rule works great if the child's sensory and oral motor system is capable of one bite. It's a hierarchy of skills," said Melanie Potock, feeding therapist and coauthor of *Raising a Happy, Healthy Eater*, "so the more sensitive kid isn't capable of taking one bite. Maybe for him, one lick might have been an option. It all depends on the child's level of comfort. One step at a time, he will eventually get there, but we venture on this journey gently and make it fun."

Eating is not a two-step process (sit down, put food in mouth) for children, the way many parents believe, explained Kay Toomey, PhD, introduced in Chapter 1. Learning to eat is actually quite complex with a steep learning curve. Pickier children, who tend to be more sensitive to food textures, may need as many as 32 steps before they are ready to put a food in their mouth!

The temperament of your child also makes a big difference. Some are more adventurous and easygoing, while others are stubborn and take a longer time to learn to like a variety of foods. Instead of jumping to that bite, Toomey suggests parents use a learning plate. When a child doesn't want a food on his plate, put a small plate nearby and ask the child to learn about the food: name it, touch it, smell it, or even kiss it. This worked wonders for my daughter as it gave her time to warm up to food and planted the seed that eating is a learned skill.

FOOD REGULATION IS IMPORTANT NO MATTER WHAT YOUR CHILD'S SIZE

Jessica recalls being obsessed with getting food into her daughter as a toddler. She was always afraid she wasn't eating enough. Once her child was school-age, though, she started to eat a lot. Jessica looked back and realized her mistake; she should have trusted her child's small appetite when she was little. Now her daughter has trouble recognizing feelings of hunger and fullness, and tends to overeat. With picky kids, overeating is often the last thing parents think about, but we need to remind ourselves about what we are teaching our kids when we ask them to eat beyond fullness. Only they know how their body feels and how food tastes in their mouth.

A better approach is to ask children to listen to their tummy. When a child says she's done, remind her to tune in and let her know when the next meal will be (for example, "Make sure you filled your tummy, we're not eating until dinnertime,"). You will be doing your child a lifetime of good by letting her manage her hunger and food intake now, so she becomes an adult who does the same.

FOOD EXPLORATION BEFORE MANNERS

We all want to teach our kids table manners, but this can get in the way of learning to eat food. For example, my daughter would never have started eating lasagna had she not been able to take the pasta pieces off and eat them separately. This is also how she started eating chicken noodle soup: she scooped out the chicken and the noodles.

When you let children pick out food and eat meals in a way that suits them, it allows them to slowly get a taste for it. This doesn't mean you don't teach them manners like saying, "No, thank you," and "please," and learning to sit quietly. But when it comes to warming up to food, don't be afraid of letting them get their hands dirty.

Yet touching and exploring food doesn't always have to be about eating. "Use food for other purposes than eating to increase the child's exposure to the food in fun, interactive ways," said Potock. "For example, learning to match colors with orange carrots and red bell peppers gets those nutritious foods in your child's hands, and that's a safe, fun place to start!"

Food exploration also extends to meal preparation. Julie Negrin, MS, certified nutritionist and author of *How to Cook with Kids,* knows that getting kids involved in the kitchen can transform their relationship with food. She says that because kids feel little control over their day-to-day environment, helping with meals gives children a sense of ownership. "I encourage parents to have kids pick out new vegetables at the market or flip through cookbooks for menu ideas," she said. "Kids have been helping with meal preparation in almost every culture for thousands of years. It's how they find their place in the 'tribe' and the world around them."

Getting kids to help in the kitchen gives them the ultimate exposure to food and what goes into each dish. Make it a regular habit to make kids part of this important process, and over time, their skills will improve. Pickier kids probably won't eat what they help make for a while, but that doesn't mean important learning and exposure isn't happening.

The Reward Dilemma

Many parents wonder if using rewards to get their child to eat is harmful or helpful. In a 2011 review, Lucy Cooke and colleagues reviewed the evidence regarding rewards and food acceptance in children.[6] The first studies, from the 1980s, revealed a backfiring effect: rewards caused decreased liking and intake of relatively palatable foods like fruit-based drinks. In some studies, when food was used as the reward, it did not increase liking for the target food, but it did increase liking for the reward food. In other words, using dessert as a reward only makes it more desirable and the healthy food less desirable.

More recent research indicates that nonfood rewards can lead to increased intake of less-palatable foods like vegetables. Some of the most promising studies utilize repeated exposure and small tastings in young children. For example, one study divided four- to six-year-olds into separate groups with one group receiving exposure with a tangible reward (like a sticker), another group receiving exposure with a verbal reward, and a third group receiving exposure without a reward. Each group was exposed to a target vegetable for twelve days. After the intervention, liking increased in all three groups, but intake only increased in the reward groups, a finding that was maintained for three months after the study.[7] Two other studies in which parents administered these experiments at home show similar results.[8,9]

What about older children? Researchers from Brigham Young University and Cornell University used money to incentivize kids to eat fruits and vegetables, resulting in significantly increased intake (80 percent). But when the monetary reward went away, consumption returned to its prior level.[10] Studies using rewards as part of the United

Kingdom's Food Dude program at schools reveal increases in healthy food intake as well. When researchers examined how this translates to eating at home, they found that while intake was higher at three months, by one year the effect was no longer seen.[11]

Other (nonfood) research on rewards show that they can undermine intrinsic motivation, which is defined as the pleasure one gets for doing a task.[12,13,14] For example, when people feel like they are being controlled, rewards decrease autonomy and competence. Some come to value the reward more than the activity itself, so when the reward goes away, so does the behavior. In other cases, especially when there is low intrinsic motivation to begin with, rewards can create interest and behavior change. While some experts say controlling rewards can "crowd out" intrinsic motivation, rewards viewed as supportive may "crowd in" intrinsic motivation.[15] Below is a summary of instances where rewards are more likely to work and not work:

Rewarding Kids	
Likely to be ineffective:	**May help:**
• Already motivated or interested in task	• Activities where there is little interest
• Use of vague performance objectives	• Use of specific performance objectives
• Rewards become expected and are promised ahead of time	• Rewards are given after desired behavior
• Rewards feel controlling	• Rewards feel supportive
• Over-reliance on rewards to change behavior	• Judiciously using rewards

Anyone considering or currently using rewards to encourage kids' healthy eating needs to weigh the pros and cons. Will it undermine a child's internal motivation to make good choices now or in the future? Or will it give the child the (friendly) push she needs?

I personally do not use rewards with my children, but I understand if this is an area you want to explore. For more on how to use nonfood rewards as outlined in the aforementioned studies, go to http://www.weightconcern.org.uk/tinytastes.

WHAT TO EXPECT

Will changing from picky to powerful feeding strategies cause your child to bloom overnight? Well, it depends. Some kids may eat better once they have structure and have more of an appetite at meals, while others take more time. Less pressure may mean one kid blooms with food exploration, while another acts out for a time with more freedom.

Even though change in terms of eating behavior does not always come quickly, there are tangible daily benefits like happier meals and more connection at the table. See how transformative it can be to accept your little guy or gal as they are. Without the agenda of getting him or her to eat, everyone is happier and eating will improve over time.

Most importantly, having the right soil, seeds, water, and sunlight will help your child bloom the way nature intended. What makes a world of difference is learning how to meet your child's nutritional needs despite erratic eating. This is what the next chapter is all about!

Chapter 6

FROM PANIC TO NUTRITION KNOW-HOW

After running a kids' nutrition series on my blog, Liisa felt better. "Thank you so much for this information on nutrition," she said. "It confirms that I'm probably doing an okay job of at least meeting the nutritional needs of my very picky, sweet-toothed four-year-old."

Although I often compare eating to other learned skills like reading and writing, I know it is different. Food is always different. The reason it is different is because children need to eat to be healthy and grow. It's hard to be patient with your child's eating when you imagine them not growing right or missing out on some vital nutrient. This chapter is all about calming the worry I know (firsthand!) most of you go through. Here, we delve into what it really takes to meet your child's nutritional needs when they don't eat perfectly.

First, some good news. According to a study published

in the *Journal of Pediatrics*, children between the ages of two and eight are the least likely to fall short on key nutrients.[1] The reason is that young children don't need as much food as parents think. The key is to avoid grazing on food and caloric drinks between meals, which fills up their little bellies (about the size of a fist), making children less hungry at mealtime.

MAGICAL FOOD GROUPS

Nutritionists set up food guides with nutrient needs in mind. Table 6.1 displays food groups, the appropriate starter portion size, and the number of daily servings that kids generally need to meet their nutritional needs.[2]

Table 6.1 Food Groups

Food Groups	Portion, Age 2–3	Daily	Portion, Age 4–8	Daily	Portion, Age 9–12	Daily
Milk, yogurt and cheese	½ cup	2 cups	½ to ¾ cup	2–3 cups	½ to 1 cup	3 cups
Protein Foods*	1 oz	2 oz	1–2 oz	3–4 oz	2 oz	5 oz
Veggies	2–3 Tbsp cooked or a few pieces raw	1 cup	3–4 Tbsp cooked or a few pieces raw	1½ cups	¼ to ½ cup or several pieces raw	2 cups

Fruit	½–1 small piece, 2–4 Tbsp canned, or 3–4 oz juice	1 cup	½–1 small piece, 4–6 Tbsp canned, or 4 oz juice	1 cup	1 cup 1 medium piece, ¼–½ cup canned, or 4 oz juice	1.5 cups
Grains	½–1 slice bread, ¼–½ cup cooked cereal, or ½–1 cup dry cereal	3 oz	1 slice bread, ½ cup cooked cereal, or 1 cup dry cereal	4 oz	1 slice bread, ½–1 cup cooked cereal, or 1 cup dry cereal	5 oz

Adapted from The Pediatric Nutrition Handbook (2008) *You can substitute 1 oz meat, fish, or poultry with 1 egg, 1 tablespoon of peanut butter, or ¼ cup cooked beans.

This all looks great, but what happens when children skip or skimp on entire food groups? I think you'll find the task of meeting your (imperfect) child's nutritional needs easier than you imagined, especially after reading the following real-life case studies.

CASE STUDY 1: SHUNNING MEAT

Shannon* was worried that her four-year-old son, Jack,* didn't eat many high-protein foods besides cheese, milk, and hot dogs. He was also lacking a bit in the fruit and vegetable department, and refused to take supplements.

Summary of Eating: Breakfast is 1–2 bowls of cereal (sometimes fortified, sometimes not) with milk. Lunch is one slice of whole-wheat bread with mayo and a slice of cheese, sometimes avocado, with fruit like applesauce, grapes, or melon, and a cup of whole milk.

Jack will only eat dinner if it's quesadillas, hot dogs, macaroni and cheese, or breakfast for dinner (pancakes or French toast). He will sometimes eat canned green beans, corn, cucumber, and carrots. For snacks, he gets Trader Joe's cereal bars, veggie straws, yogurt, graham crackers, and pretzels.

Nutrition Assessment: On days when Jack eats fortified cereal, he meets most of his nutritional needs except vitamin D (33 percent of needs) and potassium (34 percent of needs), and he is low on fiber. On a good food day with no cereal, he is still low on vitamin D and potassium, but also iron (50 percent of needs). He's getting enough protein, as his minimum needs are 19g, and he's consuming 30–50g!

Recommendations:
- Use accepted meals to introduce protein sources like mashed beans in a quesadilla and tuna or peas in the mac and cheese. Keep exposing him to different protein sources without pressuring him.
- Serve fruits and vegetables with most meals and snacks to increase his exposure and increase fiber and potassium intake. Because he accepts fruit more than veggies, vary the fruit (see Nutrition Tips at the end of the chapter for sources of vitamins A and C) and always include a bowl at dinner. Try smoothies to boost fruit and vegetable consumption.
- Add a liquid vitamin D supplement to his milk, keeping in mind the recommended daily amount is 600 International Units (IU). Provide fortified cereal every other day to meet his iron needs. He doesn't need a multivitamin if he's consuming fortified cereal (he

would get excess nutrients, especially for folic acid and vitamin A, if he gets both).

CASE STUDY 2: NO MILK

Laura wrote to me about her three-year-old daughter, Emily, who skips milk but will eat some yogurt and cheese. She was worried about her child's calcium intake.

Summary of eating: Emily eats a decent variety of food except she stopped drinking milk when she outgrew her sippy cup. She will eat cheese in a sandwich and only eats a few spoonfuls of yogurt. She also eats some fortified foods with calcium.

Nutrition Assessment: The recommended amount of calcium for three-year-olds is 700 milligrams (mg). In a typical day she is getting about 500mg, just shy of recommendations. Remember that the Daily Value (DV) for calcium is 1000mg (what most adults need), so if a food product contains 30% DV, a serving contains 300mg.

Recommendations:
- Continue to offer dairy such as milk, yogurt, and cheese at meals, as her food preferences are likely to change.
- Try smoothies made with milk, yogurt, soy beverages, tofu, and fruit/veggies. Also include cereal fortified with calcium as a snack.
- Incorporate fortified orange juice and desserts with dairy like homemade pudding. Add a vitamin D supplement daily as fortified milk and milk alternatives are a key source.

CASE STUDY 3: NO VEGGIES

Jackie emailed me about her sixteen-month-old son,

Charlie, who eats a variety of foods except for vegetables.

Summary of Eating: Breakfast is usually two 3-inch pumpkin pancakes, ⅓ cup of fruit (pears, watermelon, or applesauce) and ½ cup of milk. The mid-morning snack is a whole-wheat blueberry muffin (½ of a regular muffin or 2 mini muffins) and ½ cup of milk.

Lunch is two chicken meatballs made with basil and sundried tomatoes, ½ slice of whole-wheat bread, mixed veggies (which are refused), ⅓ cup of diced fruit or applesauce, and ½ cup of milk. The afternoon snack is a homemade smoothie with whole-milk yogurt and puréed fruit.

Dinner is the toughest meal because there are only select items Charlie will eat such as a quesadilla made with a whole-wheat tortilla, mozzarella cheese, mashed black beans, diced fruit, and sometimes yogurt for dessert and milk.

Nutrition Assessment: Charlie has no trouble meeting his vitamin and minerals needs with the variety of food he is eating. Like everyone who relies on vitamin D from their diet, he is only getting 30 percent of the DV. Another potential problem is that he is borderline low in iron (80 percent of needs), a big nutrient to watch at this age.

Recommendations:
- Include iron-rich foods such as iron-fortified cereals (good for snacks), raisins, soybeans, beans, meat, and shrimp. Give him a vitamin D supplement (RDA is 600 IU). Keep offering veggies.
- Try smoothies with greens added to them and continue to vary the fruit with meals.
- Try to eat the same meal at dinner at least a few times

per week. Rotate meals he likes with ones he doesn't. On the nights when it's a meal that he usually doesn't eat, provide one or two sides he accepts. When serving a meal he's likely to accept, provide sides that are new. He needs the exposure to start trying different foods.

*All of the names in the case studies have been changed to protect privacy.

10 TOP NUTRITION POINTS

When helping children meet nutrition needs, keep the following points in mind:

1. It's normal for young children to skimp on certain food groups, but it's still relatively easy to meet their nutritional needs. Remember that how they eat over time is what matters, not just one day or even a bad week.
2. Be aware of your child's eating pattern. Are they hungriest at breakfast or lunch? That might be the best time to bulk up on nutrition. For example, a four-year-old needs three ounces of protein. Two eggs (or two slices of French toast) in the morning and one tablespoon of peanut butter at lunch gets him there.
3. Try not to leave the most nutritious foods for the end of the day (dinner) when children are tired and don't eat as well. Offer fruits and veggies all day along with the other food groups, so you can relax at dinner and make it about family time.
4. Children do not have to eat vegetables to meet their needs. A variety of fruits, especially those with vitamin A, can get them by. To optimize nutrition, serve at least one source of vitamin C (citrus fruits, 100 percent juice,

kiwi, strawberries, broccoli, mango and red peppers) and vitamin A (sweet potato, carrots, spinach, cantaloupe, apricots, mango, and peppers) daily.

5. Young children like to "food jag," meaning they prefer to eat the same one or two foods for a period of time. A good strategy is to allow kids to enjoy their favorite foods when you serve them, but not to serve them at every meal.

6. If your child doesn't eat fish, consider fish oil supplements to ensure they get adequate amounts of the essential fatty acids docosahexaenoic acid (DHA) and eicosapentaenoic acid (EPA). International recommendations for two- to four-year-olds is 100-150mg (DHA and EPA combined), four- to six-year-olds, 150-200mg, six- to ten-year olds, 200-250mg, and ten- to eighteen-year-olds, 250-500mg.[3]

7. If your child eats more than the recommended amounts of food groups listed in the aforementioned chart, don't worry. Just make sure they eat at the table and until they are full. Appetites and amounts eaten vary greatly among kids.

8. If your child gets fortified food throughout the week (from cereal, cereal/granola bars, waffles, drinks and snack foods), a multivitamin is not needed. Children who eat poorly with few fortified foods, who are underweight, or those on a restricted diet (including strict vegetarians) or have certain medical conditions may benefit from a multivitamin.

9. If you decide against the multivitamin, taking a separate vitamin D supplement makes sense (the AAP recommends 400 IU, but new DRIs are set at 600 IU).[4]

10. For more detailed nutrition at each stage, check out my book *Fearless Feeding*.

NUTRITION CONFIDENCE

So there you have it: easy ways to meet your child's nutritional needs. Next, we focus on recipes and food strategies for the powerful kid!

PART III: THE KNOW-HOW

"The right thing to do and the hard thing to do are usually the same thing."

– Steve Maraboli

Chapter 7

FROM RANDOM TO STRATEGIC MEALS & RECIPES

You now have a new mindset about picky eating and some solid strategies to keep you going. I'm going to be honest with you—you need something more. That's because the road to feeding picky eaters is full of unexpected landmines, sharp turns, and ups and downs. In other words, it is not always easy to stay the course. You will be tempted to control your child's food intake, give up, and do all the things you know won't be good for your child over the long haul.

This last section of the book is all about the know-how that makes a huge difference. Think of it as parenting secrets that spark motivation and bring you much-needed peace of mind. This chapter focuses on the child-friendly recipes and meal ideas every parent needs in their back pocket.

FOOD STRATEGIES BY FOOD GROUP

I always laugh when I see a recipe or cookbook for the
picky kid. I think, which picky child? Every child has
different things they will eat. How does this cook know
what will be enticing to my child? (They don't, and no,
their kid is not picky after you read about what he will eat.)

That's why I go through each food group below and
discuss different ways to introduce foods to your child
followed by several recipes. This is to give you ideas; only
you know your kid and your cooking style.

FRUITS AND VEGETABLES

Avoid sneaking fruits and veggies into your child's diet;
this sends the message that these foods are so bad they
need to be hidden. Instead, show your child the numerous
ways veggies and fruits can bring life to food, and she will
start to look at them in a positive light.

- *Try different preparation methods:* Have your kids
  help you make zucchini and carrot muffins or breads,
  their favorite smoothie with leafy greens thrown in, or
  mixing the veggies in oil before roasting them. Roasting
  naturally brings out the sweetness in vegetables, which
  may be pleasing to kids.
- *Serve raw veggies with dips:* This strategy works well
  to increase intake, according to a 2012 study published
  in the *Journal of the Academy of Nutrition and
  Dietetics.* Preschoolers ate 80 percent more broccoli
  over seven weeks when they were offered with ranch
  dressing as a dip.[1]
- *Serve salads with dressing on the side:* Kids can
  choose the dressing they enjoy. You can also designate
  "salad bar" night and have kids make their own with

options like beans, different vegetables, cheese, and fruit to make it a more well-rounded meal.

- *Try veggie soup:* In *French Kids Eat Everything,* Karen Le Billon gives her kids puréed veggie soup to spark their interest in vegetables.[2] This is great in the winter, and tasting is more likely when accompanied with a straw. Once a child likes the soup, ask if they want it chunkier and gradually add some texture to it.
- *Go for the crunch:* It's not always the taste of veggies that turn kids off: it's the texture. Researchers provided kids (ages four to twelve) with carrots and green beans that were steamed, mashed, grilled, boiled, and deep-fried.[3] The kids preferred the boiled and steamed versions. Why? Because they were crunchier, had little browning, and had less of a granular texture. Experiment with different crunchy textures and see how it goes.
- *Serve fruits and veggies first:* According to a 2010 study published in the *American Journal of Clinical Nutrition,* preschoolers served bigger portions of vegetables as a first course ate 47 percent more.[4] If you put out the fruits and veggies while you're cooking, your kids might eat a whole serving of fruits and vegetables and then some. Add a tasty dip and they will eat even more.

DAIRY AND NONDAIRY

Dairy and fortified nondairy foods are good sources of calcium and other nutrients. If your child's diet is low on dairy foods, below are some ways to add them back in.

- Cheese on a sandwich (grilled or plain)
- Adding cheese to scrambled eggs
- Graham crackers dipped in yogurt

- Frozen yogurt tubes
- Homemade chocolate milk or hot chocolate
- Fruit smoothies made with yogurt or milk
- Shakes made with ice cream, milk, and ice

HIGH-PROTEIN FOODS

Young children tend to shun meat in favor of starchy carbs. The good news is that most kids get enough protein, but nutrients in high-protein foods (like iron and zinc) and protein's filling factor can be missing.

- Add breading to typical protein sources such as fish and chicken (see recipe).
- Introduce eggs via tasty French toast sprinkled with cinnamon .
- Add protein (beans, chicken, etc.) in very small amounts to favorite quesadillas and burritos.
- Pan fry proteins (to make crispy) versus baking; once accepted, try the item baked.

WHOLE GRAINS

The general guidance for whole grains is to serve them at least half the time. Some sources are obvious, like using whole-wheat bread, whole oats in baked goods, and serving dishes with brown rice. Sometimes we need to get acceptance of an item first before jumping into whole-grain territory.

- Try white rice first if your child is more likely to try it. Once she accepts it, tell her you are going to try brown rice instead. Same goes for pasta and bread. Add whole-wheat flour or oats to muffins, pancakes, and breads.
- Use a similar sauce for grain dishes but change the

grain (for example, if your child likes the rice dish you prepare, use the same sauce when making quinoa).

- Try small amounts of oatmeal with your child's favorite dry cereal and slowly change the proportions.

FATS

Fat is an important source of nutrition for growing kids because it's rich in calories. Healthy fats that come from plants like olive oil, nuts and seeds, and avocado are sources of vitamin E, a nutrient in which many kids' diets fall short.[5] While animal fats are fine, research favors vegetable fats in terms of long-term health benefits.[6]

- Brush homemade pizza dough with some olive oil and garlic before adding toppings.
- Offer nuts with snacks and spread nut butters on toast.
- Offer nut butters to use for dipping fruits like apples.
- Use avocados to make guacamole to have with tortilla chips.
- Make your own trail mix by mixing nuts, whole-grain cereal, dried fruit, and sweet items like chocolate chips.
- Build on a grilled cheese sandwich by gradually adding avocado and other thin slices of vegetables.

RECIPES

Fruit and Veggie Muffins

Ingredients:
- 1 cup mashed moist fruit or veggie (banana, apple-sauce, cooked pumpkin, or butternut squash)
- 1 cup grated dry veggie (zucchini or carrots)
- ¼ cup brown sugar (unpacked)
- 2 eggs

- 2 teaspoons cinnamon
- ¼ teaspoon nutmeg
- ¼ teaspoon salt
- 1 cup quick-cooking rolled oats
- 1 cup flour (can use white or whole-wheat pastry flour)
- 1 teaspoon baking powder
- ½ teaspoon baking soda
- milk (only to thin out if needed)

Instructions:
1. Preheat oven to 350 degrees. Place mashed fruit and grated veggie in a medium bowl along with the brown sugar, eggs, cinnamon, nutmeg, and salt. Mix until well combined.
2. In a separate bowl, add the dry ingredients (oats, flour, baking powder, and baking soda). Add the dry ingredients to the wet ingredients and mix. Gradually add milk if the batter is too think.
3. Pour muffin batter into greased muffin tins and bake for 20–22 minutes or until a toothpick inserted into the batter comes out clean.

Chocolate Peanut Butter Smoothie*

Ingredients:
- 1 small or ½ large banana
- ½ cup frozen blueberries
- ½ apple or pear
- 1 cup spinach
- 1 celery stick, chopped
- 2 tablespoons all-natural peanut butter
- 1 tablespoon unsweetened cocoa powder
- 1 cup milk

- ½ cup ice

Instructions:
1. Mix all ingredients in a blender until smooth. Makes 3 cups.

*To make a sweeter smoothie, replace the apple or pear with strawberries, omit the peanut butter and add ½ cup plain yogurt and ½ cup orange juice in place of the milk. Skip the celery if you are not using a high-powered blender.

White Bean Banana Bread

Ingredients:
- 1 cup white flour
- 1 cup whole-wheat pastry flour
- 2 teaspoons baking powder
- ½ teaspoon baking soda
- 1 cup mashed white beans
- 1 cup mashed banana
- 1 teaspoon vanilla
- 1 teaspoon cinnamon
- ⅓ cup brown sugar (not packed)
- ¼ cup canola oil
- ¼ cup applesauce
- 2 eggs

Instructions:
1. Preheat oven to 350 F. In a medium bowl, add both types of flour and the baking powder and soda and set aside.
2. In a large mixing bowl, add the beans and mash with a fork until mashed together. Add the bananas and

continue to mash mixing the two together. Add in vanilla, cinnamon, brown sugar, canola oil, applesauce and eggs and mix well.

3. Once mixed, add the dry ingredients and continue to mix with a spoon until it makes a consistent batter.

4. Spray a 9x5 loaf pan with cooking spray and add the batter. Cook in the oven for about 50 minutes or until a toothpick comes out clean. Let it cool 15 minutes before serving.

Chicken Tenders (Adapted from *Fearless Feeding*)

Ingredients:
- ¾ cup bread crumbs
- ¼ cup parmesan cheese, finely grated
- ½ teaspoon salt
- ½ teaspoon paprika
- ½ teaspoon garlic powder
- ½ teaspoon mustard powder
- Butter, melted or egg, beaten
- 1 lb chicken or fish, cut into small pieces

Instructions:
1. Preheat oven to 400F.
2. Combine the first six ingredients in a medium bowl.
3. Melt butter or beat the egg in another bowl.
4. Dip chicken or fish in butter or egg and dredge through bread crumb mixture.
5. Cook chicken 20-22 minutes and fish 8-10 minutes or until done.

Fried Rice

Ingredients:
- 2 garlic cloves, minced
- 1 tablespoon oil
- ¾ cup frozen peas and carrots, thawed
- 2 eggs
- 2 cups cooked brown or white rice
- 1 tablespoon soy sauce
- 1 tablespoon oyster sauce

Instructions:
1. Scramble eggs and set aside.
2. Add oil, garlic, and thawed veggies to heated skillet.
3. Mix until heated and well combined. Combine cooked brown rice, eggs, and sauce with veggies.

Coconut-Butternut Squash Crockpot Soup (Courtesy of *Super Healthy Kids*)

Ingredients:
- 3 cups butternut squash, chopped
- 3 cups chopped sweet potato
- 1 onion, chopped
- 2 cups chicken broth
- ¼ cup butter
- 2 cups half and half (or coconut milk)
- ½ teaspoon cumin
- 2 tablespoons shredded coconut

Instructions:
1. Place squash, sweet potato, onion, 1 cup of chicken broth and butter in a slow cooker, and cook on high for about 4 hours.

2. Using an immersion blender, or scooping your squash into a regular blender, puree until smooth.
3. Return to slow cooker and add remaining chicken broth, half and half, cumin, and coconut.
4. Cook for about 30 more minutes, or until soup is heated through. Sprinkle with extra coconut for garnishing.

HAPPY COOKING

I hope this chapter has inspired you to creatively add nutritious foods to your child's diet. Remember this is a process that takes time, but it's well worth it.

Chapter 8

FROM HANDS OFF TO HANDS ON

When my son was in kindergarten, he had a hard time keeping up. The class always seemed to move on before he had mastered the material. He was still trying to sound out letters, for example, while everyone else was sounding out words. By the end of the year, he was very much behind and acting out. Knowing he had trouble learning, along with language delays, we put him in a summer learning program at Lindamood-Bell.

People with a learning disability like my son (we had him tested the following year), really just learn differently. They are usually of average or above-average intelligence, but need to be taught in a systematic way that breaks material down into smaller parts and gives ample time for practice. Multisensory teaching is also beneficial instead of the typical auditory-focused lessons. For example, these kids benefit from using all of their senses such as visual aids, touching (kinesthetic), and movement to learn new material. His time at Lindamood-Bell was individualized and gave him what he needed to learn how to read.

You can think of children and food the same way as you think of children and learning. Cautious eaters need more exposure and practice than kids who take to food more easily. They benefit from learning about different food groups and how meals are put together (especially mixed dishes, which freak them out!). For example, when I offered my son an egg sandwich, something he typically turned down, I instead tried the learning approach. He already liked eggs and English muffins, but he just didn't realize it was the same thing because it looked different. So I brought him in the kitchen and explained what I was doing: "Instead of scrambling the egg, I'm going to pan fry it." He saw me make it step by step, and when the sandwich was done, he sat down and ate the whole thing.

But if I had just made it privately and then served it to him, he would have never eaten it. Going that extra step of explaining and showing picky eaters the ins and outs of food helps a great deal. A more adventurous kid might be fine being served an egg sandwich, but a cautious eater will see it as "different" and refuse to eat it.

LEARNING ABOUT FOOD

This chapter is about the hands-on experience kids need but don't always get with food. The problem is picky eaters are typically offered fewer opportunities in the kitchen than more adventurous eaters, even though they need it more. No doubt, they can be resistant, but once the habit and traditions are set, they usually learn to love it. Best of all, your child will begin to see food in a whole new light.

There are many ways you can take this learning approach with your child. Here are some tips:

- Don't make the agenda be about tasting or eating food.

Make the agenda about food learning.

- Teach children all the different food items that go into meals introducing them one at a time (grains, fruits, vegetables, dairy, proteins, fats, herbs and spices, and condiments). Explain the different ways these items can be prepared and combined to make food yummy and satisfying. Allow touching and tasting if the child wants.

- Explain meal prep while cooking. Show your child what is going into the meal and why. Visit farmers markets, farms, or plant a garden to show children how food is grown.

- Plan restaurant adventure nights every month or so to introduce different foods to kids. Educate your child on the foods they can expect to see before going. Look up pictures on the Internet and watch some videos on YouTube.

- Teach children how to anticipate the texture of different foods. For younger picky eaters, texture is often what turns kids off instead of taste. Show kids how they can anticipate the texture of food by touching it, and explain textures before eating when you can.

- Show children how to taste a food by taking a very small piece and placing it on the tongue, taking it out if they wish.

The more kids learn about food, the more comfortable they will become around food. Think of it as turning up food exposure a major notch! It also gives you a dialogue around meals. For example, if you are eating at a friend's house and they are serving a mixed dish, you can explain that it has a grain (rice), dairy (cheese), vegetable (carrots) and protein (chicken), all items you have introduced and talked about.

The next very important step to hands-on learning is teaching kids some basic cooking skills.

COOKING

Research shows that children who cook eat a wider variety of foods than those who don't.[1] But I think this message of "cooking to eat" is not a helpful one. That's because when kids cook and don't eat the food or meal, parents see it as a failure and may stop bringing their child into the kitchen. Again, coming around to food takes longer for cautious eaters but they are learning a valuable skill they'll use for a lifetime. I believe every parent needs to teach kids how to cook before they grow up and leave home.

Teaching my kids to cook got off to a rocky start, and still can be challenging at times. "You want to help with dinner?" I'd ask. They'd politely respond with "No thank you." Not wanting to force them, I let it go. Also, once they started school and had homework, I didn't want to bog them down with more things to do. But soon I realized I was approaching it all wrong. I needed to create structure and habit around teaching them to cook, and that's exactly what I did.

In my book *What to Cook for Dinner with Kids,* I show parents how to develop core rotation of dinner meals. As part of that, I include specific cooking jobs for kids. One of the rules in my house is each kid gets one small job with dinner. It might be a simple task, like washing veggies, or helping set the table. As part of those weekly chores, I also put each kid on dinner duty at least once a week. They are my little helpers throughout the whole meal (even when they run off — and I have to pull them back in).

Each week I have a "kids' choice" night where the kids can choose the dinner meal. But I transitioned it from kids' choice, to kids' choice *and* make. I'm no longer getting the ingredients for them either—they have to do it all, start to finish. I'm there to help but not lead (with a glass of wine in hand — after all, it's my night off!).

The key is to start slow and gradually add on cooking jobs. You may get off track when things get busy but just keep at it. Summer is also a more relaxed time to have cooking adventures with your kids. If you don't know how to cook, consider taking a cooking class together. No doubt it takes effort, but seeing your child thriving in the kitchen will be worth it.

Kitchen Independence

In the book *How to Raise an Adult*, Julie Lythcott-Haims details how parents today do way too much for their kids. There are various reasons for this, including nonstop extracurricular activities and school work. The problem is that when kids leave home, they know how to get an A on a test and kick a soccer ball, but lack the vital life skills they will need to use every day.[2] So in addition to cooking, you also want to teach kids how to be independent in the kitchen. Following are three easy ways to get started with kitchen independence.

Make Tableware Accessible
It dawned me that while I'm cooking dinner, I hand my kids plates to set the table. That's because they cannot reach the plates and cups – and if they use a stool they get in my way. So I changed things around and put plates, cups, and bowls in the lower cabinet, making them easier for the kids to reach. Here are some things they can do as a result of this simple change:

- Set the table by themselves from start to finish
- Help unload the dishwasher
- Get water/drinks for themselves

ORGANIZE YOUR KITCHEN WITH KIDS IN MIND
I organized my kitchen so it's easier to teach my children about food. For example, I arrange my cabinets by food groups: grains (bread, crackers, and rice/other dry grains), protein (beans, nuts, and canned fish), fruits and veggies (canned veggies/tomatoes, and dried fruit) and goodies (chocolate or anything sweet). Older children can help make grocery lists by looking through the cabinets to see what is needed. It helps to have printed lists on cabinets with what needs to be stocked.

CUT, POUR, AND SERVE THEMSELVES
I realized that I was still cutting my kids' meat and pouring their milk (those big jugs are heavy!). Yeah, they might spill but isn't that how they learn how to handle it better next time? Now they are doing all these things themselves, with guidance from me. In *How to Raise an Adult,* Lythcott-Haims recommends this easy strategy for teaching kids any new skill:

- *Watch me do it:* Have children watch you once or twice, explaining how you do it
- *Let's do it together:* Assist them a few times
- *I watch you do it:* Watch and provide feedback until they can do it independently

EVERYBODY BENEFITS FROM GETTING INVOLVED WITH FOOD

Kids are taught certain core subjects in school. They need

to learn to read and write, for example, and will use this skill no matter what they choose as a career. They may not become professional writers, but communicating through the written word is essential. Everyone also needs to learn about food from what it is, to forming a meal, to shopping and cooking. We all have to eat to live, so cooking is a non-negotiable task.

This doesn't mean children need to become foodies or love to cook the way a chef does. They just need to find a way to make some basic meals that taste good and are nutritious. Too often, picky eaters are labeled as not being interested in food, so they stay far away from the kitchen. But they need this exposure even more because a child that is naturally drawn to food is more likely to seek those experiences. As parents, we have to try even harder with the slow-to-warm-up kids. But they all benefit, no matter what their eating personality.

Does giving your picky eater hands-on experience with food mean they will branch out? Over the long haul, I'd say yes; but focusing on this outcome only hurts the process. Learning about food and cooking can only help, even when kids remain resistant. Giving your child hands-on experience with food now is something that will eventually pay off, in more ways than you can imagine.

Next, some inspiration straight from the pages of my blog.

Chapter 9

FROM NEEDING TO KNOW TO HAVING FAITH

Since first publishing *From Picky to Powerful* as an e-book in 2014, I have added several posts on picky eating to my blog. I wanted to include these posts in the latest edition of the book. These posts bring up some important points you may not have thought of before—just more picky eater food for thought.

WANT TO REFORM YOUR PICKY EATER? TAKE ADVICE FROM BUDDHA [BLOG POST]

I was reading about the latest Picky Eater Project (Can Young Picky Eaters Reform? 10 Rules, and a Plan) on the New York Times Well Family. If you're not familiar, Sally Simpson and Natalie Digate Muth help a family struggling with picky eaters. A lot of the rules they put in place are sound and familiar: eat one meal; keep it pleasant; have something at the table kids prefer; get them cooking, etc.[1]

After reading the article, I peeked at the comments. Quite a few parents wrote about how they do all these things and their kid still isn't branching out. And I realize the thing that is happening is the thing that is *always* happening. It's what makes feeding kids really, really hard.

OUR ATTACHMENT TO OUTCOMES

Let's say you have a family, two parents and a five-year-old who aren't having family dinners. Instead, the parents opt to feed their picky son his own meal and then make their own later. When they finally switch to family dinners, they're disappointed that their son still has a limited menu. After a few months, they inch their way back to the old way, figuring family dinners didn't work for them.

The problem isn't that family meals weren't effective, it's that the parents were only focused on one outcome: *the child eating more foods*. Buddha says all suffering is due to attachment, something I see happen with kids' eating all the time.

THIS TUNNEL VISION MAKES IT HARD TO SEE PROGRESS

When we are focused on a desired outcome, we fail to see other benefits that come from what we do. For the story above, the child is now eating dinner with this family without complaints. That's progress. The child is getting exposed to different foods. That's progress. The child is feeling his parents believe in him enough to invite him to eat with them. That's huge progress.

In one of the article's comments, a parent describes her child as able to cook but still unable to eat a good portion of what she makes. But a child who can cook is an awesome thing, right? I'm sure more experimentation with food will follow, as long as she is not labeled "the cook that doesn't eat."

Most importantly, when we focus solely on outcomes, we fail to address the underlying issues causing them. In this book I have used the analogy of growing a plant. You need the right soil, seeds, and water/sunlight to make a plant grow. But each plant is different; some need more water, and others need more sunlight. And some plants grow quickly, while others grow much more slowly. A plant that is slower to grow isn't a bad thing, it just might need a bit more water and time to flourish.

THE HOW: INTENTION AND ACCEPTANCE

Like any parent, I am vulnerable to this "outcome trap" too. My son can drive me crazy with his picky ways. I have found that when I find this happening (first sign: I'm miserable), I check in with my intention and how that spills over to my ability to accept his present eating or not.

Let's say I'm cooking something new and invite him in the kitchen to check it out. I tell him what it is and offer for him to help or just watch as I make it. If my intention is to teach him about food, then that's what I do. Whether he tries it or not, I'm okay with it because my intention was to teach, not to get him to eat.

But if I do the same thing with the intention of getting him to eat at dinner, he'll feel the pressure from the get-go. That's because I exaggerate how tasty the food is, giving him every opportunity to taste it. When it comes dinner time, I remind him *again* how he helped make it and when he refuses to try it at my request, I roll my eyes.

Which one do you think will have a more positive effect on his eating over time? Which one better allows me to stay the course and keep things in perspective?

I'm all for sharing stories and advice to help struggling parents, but I'm always cautious when I hear words like "reform" or "cure." Because I want parents to understand that even when they make positive changes, not all kids will react in the same way, but that doesn't mean important learning isn't going on. One child who learns to cook will want to expand his tastes while another stays cautious. Children bloom with food in their own time, so we can't stop giving them what they need to grow.

PICKY EATING: WHAT'S MISSING IN THE NATURE VERSUS NURTURE DEBATE? [BLOG POST]

I posted an article on my Facebook page (An Open Letter to the Moms Who Judged My Kids for Being Picky Eaters) and got lots of great feedback. But I soon realized that while I like the article's no-judgment message, its overall takeaway may be one of helplessness. That's because if picky eaters are born and not made, like the article says, there's not much parents can do.[2] To me, this is just as bad as choosing the other side of the argument: picky eaters are made, not born.

The problem with labeling kids' eating as *all nature* or *all nurture* is that neither is true. It's a messy combination of both. Sadly, something important gets lost every time this issue is hotly debated.

THE ALL-NATURE MISTAKE

There's little doubt that every child is born with certain food preferences, some individual to them and some based on developmental factors. One study shows that preferences for protein, vegetables and fruit tend to be more genetically influenced while snack food, starches and dairy preferences are shaped more by one's shared environment.[3] A child's reluctance to try unfamiliar food (food neophobia) peaks between two and six and is highly genetically linked.[4]

When we choose the all nature side, we risk labeling kids' eating ability way too early. This can result in short-order cooking or never offering different foods. Just because a child is cautious with food at five doesn't mean he can't learn to like different food over time. Kids are constantly changing — mind and body — but beliefs that children's eating habits are static will naturally lead to fewer opportunities for them to learn and grow with food.

THE ALL-NURTURE MISTAKE

Although parents greatly influence children's eating over time, they cannot control their food preferences, how their body turns out, or how much food they need to grow. Research shows that what mom eats during pregnancy and how and what infants are fed influences a child's food preferences.5 But doing "everything right" does not guarantee a young child who will eat everything.

When parents choose the all-nurture side, it leads to a lot of guilt and effort to raise the child who eats perfectly. This can result in tense meals and controlling feeding practices that negatively impact eating over the long haul. In some instances, kids may eat a certain way to please their parents, but rebel later or when at their friends' houses. In short, parents are trying to control what they can't because of the underlying belief that they are completely responsible for what and how much their child eats.

THE MIDDLE GROUND

My son was a bad sleeper from day one, unlike his older sister who slept through the night at four months. Having read up on sleep, I knew he had colic, and it usually improved around four months, which thankfully it did. But it wasn't until he was eighteen months that he slept most nights without waking. Even though it was obvious he wasn't sleep-trained as early as my daughter, I knew he could get there with support from us.

I think we get too hung up on kids doing things early and that gets in the way of doing our job. I didn't like that my son had trouble learning to sleep, but what good would it do to go against his nature? I could have let him "cry it out" at six months, but I know my spirited son would have been the baby who cried for four hours straight. Worse yet, I could have given up, labeling my kid as a "bad sleeper." Instead, my husband and I stayed consistent with naps and bedtimes until he seemed ready to go it alone at eighteen months.

I would never, ever judge a parent for their child's limited food choices. But I hope every parent understands how powerful they are in helping shape their child's eating — and relationship with food — over time. It shouldn't be about choosing a side but about using the knowledge of a child's *nature* to effectively *nurture* him in the best possible direction.

WHY I'M NEITHER FOR NOR AGAINST KID FOOD [BLOG POST]

Every year we go to Red Lobster for a family member's birthday. This year, my daughter announced she wanted to order lobster. I suggested we share the big lobster meal, and she agreed. I was ecstatic to find her opting out of the kids' menu.

I posted pictures on the my Facebook page, saying how I wish food on kids' menus were just smaller portions of regular menu items, and got a variety of comments:

"I agree, but I also feel like we eat at restaurants so seldom that I don't really worry about it."

"We always share the adult food, and say no to the kids' menu."

It seems some parents are strongly against "kid food" while others are okay with it. The more I thought about it, the more I realized I really don't have strong feelings either way. And here's why:

WHOSE JOB IS IT TO FEED KIDS ANYWAY?

Due to a variety of factors, family eating patterns began to change around the 1970s. Frozen dinners and other convenience foods popped up everywhere, and eating out grew from an occasional outing to a regular occurrence. According to the 2015 Dietary Guidelines Report, in the late 1970s about 18 percent of calories were consumed away from home but by 2005-2008 that number jumped to 32 percent.[6]

It's easy to blame the food industry, but the truth is they are running a business. And businesses give people what they want, not what they need. If you went to buy your umpteenth pair of black shoes, would the department store tell you "no" because you don't *really* need them? That doesn't happen! As long as there's a market for chicken nuggets, they won't go away. And if people continue to believe large portions provide value, they won't go away either.

Parents always will do a much better job of feeding their kids than a restaurant or packaged food designed for kids ever could. The problem occurs when parents allow businesses to take over this very important job. So in our house, eating out is a treat that occurs about once a week.

I REFUSE TO MAKE A BIG DEAL OUT OF THE KIDS' MENU

I'd love to say my kids have no interest in the kids' menu, but that would be a lie. My daughter loves chicken nuggets, and my son is fan of mac and cheese and burgers. I could insist they split a meal off the regular menu — forbidding the kid fare — but that would bring even more attention to kids' meals. So they get to order from them, but I do have some rules.

I simply ask that if we are at a Mexican restaurant that they order Mexican food (no burgers at a Mexican or Chinese restaurant please!). If it's the second night eating out, usually when on vacation, they need to order something different than the previous night. And if the main meal is fried, the side dish can't be fried.

Restaurants also can be a way to expand kids' tastes, especially with ethnic foods. Before going someplace new, I'll check out the restaurant's menu online to see if there's something the kids will like. For example, there's a new Thai place nearby, and I spy some noodle dishes, chicken on a stick and peanut sauce for dipping that can get the kids interested so that's on the list to try out. But when meeting family members out, we usually choose kid-friendly places where children can be loud and the typical kids' menu reigns.

Do I wish "kid food" was never invented? Definitely! But I refuse to give the topic too much of my time and energy. I'm sure my kids will eventually outgrow kid food if I do my job of exposing them to a wider variety. I just don't expect restaurants or food companies to do that for me.

WANT TO RAISE A GOOD EATER? LET YOUR CHILD MAKE THESE 3 FOOD MISTAKES [BLOG POST]

Everywhere I turn, some expert is talking about the problem of over-involved parents. A new book that was recently reviewed in The New York Times, "The Gift of Failure," explains how children are better off when they can actually make mistakes on their own. Because, well, that's how they learn.[7]

But watching a kid struggle when we know the answer — or how to do it better — isn't always easy. One area completely overlooked in this realm of failing is eating. To learn about food, eating and their body, kids need to mess up. So here are the top three "learning mistakes" I think kids need to experience.

1. LET THEM GET HUNGRY

When a child says he's hungry, it can send any adult into a panic searching for food. But what does this teach? Hunger is something that needs to be attended to immediately. Whether that's the intention or not, kids catch on that hunger is something to get rid of quick.

When my kids say they are hungry before dinner I always answer with "good, you'll enjoy the meal more." We want kids to learn that pangs of hunger do not need to be fixed immediately. When kids experience the consequence of not getting enough at meals, they are incentivized to fill up when they get the chance. And when they don't always see favorite food at gatherings — and they choose not to eat — they learn what happens: *hunger*. Putting aside medical conditions and special circumstances, the occasional longer-than-parents-like bout of hunger teaches kids how to do a better job of managing their hunger.

2. LET THEM EAT TOO MUCH

"Don't eat too much, you'll get a tummy ache." Parents often hover to make sure kids get just the right amount of sweets. But eating past fullness, especially non-nutritious items, teaches kids a few different lessons.

First, it can remove the taboo from non-nutritious foods. If my kids seem to be obsessed about some food, I plan an eat-all-you-can snack with the item. Sure enough, they stop asking for it. It squashes their curiosity instead of piquing it.

Second, they can learn the adverse effects of eating too much of food that simply isn't good at nourishing the body. My daughter now realizes that starchy foods, like Cheez-Its, don't fill her up. She learned that thanks to her weekly visit to Grandma's.

A child can only learn the limits of his body by experiencing them.

3. LET THEM COOK THEIR WAY

My daughter made guacamole from start to finish the other night with no help from me. It ended up way too watery. You better believe next time she will add less yogurt and salsa. We talked about how you can always add more so it's best to start off small.

Those nice and neat pictures of kids helping in the kitchen are not real! It gets messy, and they make mistakes. But then one time they get it right and their confidence builds. And you realize the mistakes are what taught them.

Coco, a mom of two girls six and eight, has had her kids helping in the kitchen since they were two. Now they can cook simple meals on their own. But she remembers lots of mistakes, "We once made pizza and whilst making the dough, my daughter accidentally put too much liquid into the flour and it became more like a paste," she says. "We played with the paste on the table for a while, and the pizza ended up having bread as its base."

There's a myth that good eaters always eat a variety of foods, stop after consuming balanced portions, are natural cooks, and only want one cookie (if that!). No, the kids who grow into good eaters are the ones who were allowed to make mistakes and learn from them. Of course, with supportive parents there to help guide them.

WHAT KIDS REALLY MEAN WHEN THEY SAY "I DON'T LIKE IT" [BLOG POST]

It was Cultural Heritage Day at my son's school, and for lunch parents brought in food from their nationality. As one boy sat down to his plate of unfamiliar food, he started to cry. I went up to him to see if he was okay and he said, "I don't like this food."

I went around to all the items, explaining what they were, and that helped a little. He ended up picking up a churro to eat and started to calm down.

Here's the thing: His reaction had nothing to do with not liking the food and everything to do with not feeling ready to eat it.

"I DON'T LIKE IT" OR "I'M NOT READY?"

On the blog Mealtime Hostage, Skye, the mom of a selective eater, tells amazing stories about her son's food journey. In one of her posts, her son responded with "I'm not ready" after being asked if he wanted a food.[8] Not only was this an insightful response, it reminded me what's really going on when young children say they don't like something. Basically kids are saying "This food looks too challenging to eat." It's kind of like if you were served a meal of fried insects. Would you want to dig in or get comfortable with the idea of it first?

The typical response to "I don't like it" from parents and caregivers is "How do you know, you've never tried it?" Then everyone tries to persuade the little one into eating the food by saying how good it tastes or how healthy it is. This pressure and attention actually drives the child away from the food in question. All the while, the kid's real challenge hasn't been addressed at all.

So if a child isn't ready to eat a food, the question becomes: Can parents help the child become ready?

GIVING CHILDREN THE SUPPORT THEY NEED

When a child doesn't feel ready there can be a few things going on. First, it could be, like the story above, that there is just too much unfamiliar food at once. Serving at least one thing your child is likely to accept helps them ease into positively experiencing different foods.

Another way to support your child is detailed by dietitian Sarah Remmer who blogs at the Yummy Mummy Club. After noticing her son's disinterest in dinner she started to ask him this question: "What can we do to make this meal yummier for you?" Here's what happened:

When I started asking my preschooler this question, it literally transformed our mealtimes for the better. And the answers were very interesting! One night, he asked for ketchup to dip his steamed broccoli into (after which, he gobbled it up), and another night when he said that he didn't like his chili, I asked him if grated cheese would help, which ended up being a game-changer. Your child might need some ideas from you such as "Do you need dip for your veggies?" or "Would you like me to separate your meat from your rice?" but nine times out of ten, you and your child might be able to come up with a fun way to make his meal more palatable.[9]

Sometimes children need to learn more about the food for acceptance to occur. Examples include getting involved with preparation and playing with food without being disrespectful. Parents can also warn kids about the texture and taste of something new, where the food comes from, and help them identify items that are similar to other things they eat.

Other times, children simply need time and consistent opportunities, as Amy Roskelley from the popular website Super Healthy Kids points out:

My kids used to not eat salad at all! In fact, I would serve them salad for years, only to have them take one bite just because they had to. But I didn't stop. For years and years, I didn't stop! Until one day, they just started eating salad. You know how they say it takes 8-10 exposures to a new food for a kid to try it? Try 8-10 YEARS! ... It doesn't bother me that it took so long! The bottom line is... don't be frustrated. Don't make it a big deal, and be patient!! The most important thing you can do is to continue to make vegetables the star of every meal![10]

So if your child says he doesn't like a meal, it probably means he doesn't feel ready to eat it. Whether it's additional support he needs to get over the hump, or time and repeated exposure, parents can be more effective when they address what's really going on.

BEING ABLE TO SEE WHAT OTHERS DON'T

There's more to feeding kids than just getting them to eat healthy food. Having perspective can go a long way toward staying the course, and raising your child to be the best eater he can be. In this last chapter, we have pearls of wisdom from moms who've been there, and have made it out the other side.

Chapter 10

FROM PICKY TO POWERFUL STORIES

Hearing from parents who have been there with picky eating can help a great deal. It reminds us that if we trust in the process, all will be well in the end. And, it just feels good knowing that we are not alone!

ON ADVICE YOU'D GIVE YOUR YOUNGER SELF (FROM PARENTS OF OLDER CHILDREN)

Sandy Nissenberg, MS, RD

I would tell myself not to stress about the little things, to keep good food options available, get the kids involved as much as possible, and eat together as a family. Personally, I did much of this, and although I did wonder if the picky eating phase would improve when the kids were young, I can now say I see the results. My two kids, now in their twenties, are very aware of their food intake, and both have become very physically active as well. I'm very proud of how far they have come.

Christine Columbo, RD

The advice I would give my young-mom self regarding my three picky-eater children:

- Serve the vegetables first when the children are hungry! Or serve them as a pre-dinner snack when they are willing to eat (almost) anything.
- Peer pressure works! Have them eat with other children who are more accepting of vegetables. But stay away from his friend Nick, who along with his mother, is an extremely picky eater.
- Because Daddy is a super-taster, one of you will be one, too, and will reject anything bitter. Serve those vegetables with some cheese sauce or butter to make them yummier. Make Daddy eat some, too.
- You know how those vegetables seem to have vanished? Look at the hidden shelf just below the surface of the kitchen table. That's where the peas and other veggies went.
- It will be a long wait. Each of your children quit being picky eaters just when they began high school. Don't waste your energy being frustrated.

Maureen Blight, R.D.

My top-level advice for parents of young children is to focus on the end game: by the time your child moves out of your house, they can eat a wide variety of foods from all five food groups. How much and what they eat on any particular day or week, especially when they are very young, doesn't really matter that much.

Realize that your child needs to be offered foods many times before they will try it or eat it willingly. I know research says it takes up to fifteen exposures before the "average child" will eat a new food, but my children needed much more time. Also, as a parent, it is very hard to see progress. We went camping every year with another family (a dietitian friend of mine). She commented one year that she saw a big difference in one of my son's willingness to eat different foods from the previous year, progress that I had failed to notice.

If I had the chance to do it over again, I'd introduce the concept of the "learning plate" that can hold foreign foods that your child is reluctant to try. This learning plate allows exploration without the expectation of eating. I'd also serve more unfamiliar foods to the whole family (yes, pushing my husband outside of his comfort zone), so we all experiment and expand our collective palate. Perhaps I was too busy to do this as a working mother with two sons only 19 months apart, but I'm sure I could have tried a new recipe once a month.

I can't overstate the importance of teaching good table manners. We did a pretty good job but could have done better about teaching the importance of taking smaller bites of food and not talking while chewing. Parents have the right to insist on good table manners (even the picky eaters). It is not okay for children to throw food down or say food is yucky. It is our responsibility to teach them the right words such as, "I'd like to be excused from the table now," or "Thank you for making food for me, but I don't like this."

Finally, I encourage you to include your children in food preparation as early as possible. What I didn't realize is once my children were immersed in sports, scouts, and other activities, there was no time left to teach cooking. In my case, the window of opportunity to teach cooking skills was limited to when they were pretty young. Cooking is an essential skill, so pass on your knowledge when you can. And if you don't know how to cook, it is time to explore your options to learn simple survival skills in the kitchen!

Bettina Segal, creator of The Lunch Tray blog

My twelve-year-old son, the veggie-avoider, came to me unsolicited to offer a dinner suggestion. He wanted — and I swear, this was the exact request – "Portobello mushroom burgers with Gruyere cheese and pesto aioli." So that's exactly what I made for dinner and, yes, my son enthusiastically ate every bite. But if you'd told me this story just a few years ago, I would have laughed in your face. The veggie-avoider making an entire meal of a big, black and somewhat scary-looking mushroom? Not gonna happen in this lifetime.

So here's my advice: Remember that you know your own kid better than anyone else. So if an expert says the "one-bite" rule is a terrible idea, but you suspect your child would react well to that little push, then go for it. And if another expert says the "one-bite" rule is a terrific idea, but you know it's only going to ignite an ugly mealtime battle that goes precisely nowhere, then forget it. Your intuition is worth more than the tallest stack of "expert" advice books on picky eating.

And finally, most importantly, please take the long view. It took us twelve incredibly frustrating years to get there, but now, apparently, Portobello mushroom burgers with Gruyere cheese and pesto aioli are here to stay on this family's dinner rotation.

ON FOSTERING INDEPENDENCE

Amy Roskelley, creator of Super Healthy Kids

When my son started taking a lunch to school in the first grade, I realized very quickly he wasn't eating what I packed. In fact, one day near Halloween, he told me that he traded his entire lunch for a single candy corn! (He's a very honest kid.) It was at that moment I realized no matter how healthy I wanted my kids to eat, in the end, it was up to them whether they actually ate healthy food or not.

So, I turned the lunch packing over to him. I let him make food choices, within healthy guidelines, but he packed it himself. When he chose what went in his lunch, he ate what he brought. Fast-forward to today, and that boy is in high school, and he's an amazing eater! He has packed his own lunch since the first grade, and he always brings fruits and veggies. And to my delight, he no longer trades them away!

ABOUT REALISTIC PROGRESS

Melody, mother of four

My kids were pretty resistant at first, but something you said in that first blog I read was to not quit. Keep going. Just like any other challenge in life, it's going to take more than a day. So, I got rid of all our junk food and processed food. Big mistake. I went from one extreme to another. While I knew my kids couldn't eat junk if I didn't have it around, I found that even I like to splurge now and then! I have learned to control the snack foods I have. There are lots of companies out there who make all-natural and even organic snacks. Sometimes they are a little bit pricier, but I don't mind that because our health is an investment. I read labels like crazy. I'm more in tune with how we eat than ever before. The snacks they do eat don't contain artificial colors and fake ingredients. I try very hard to always give them real food!

When my kids stopped asking for chicken nuggets, and wouldn't even eat them anymore, I knew I had made progress. When they ask me to make them a smoothie (even when carrots are inside), I know I have made progress. When we go to restaurants, we always sub fruit for fries. They don't complain. That is progress.

I think the key to helping my family was not giving up when it was really hard. We still have our trying times, but we get through them more quickly. And we definitely have less trying times. Dinner isn't always a struggle. My husband is on board, and I have learned to make a lot of new dishes that don't involve processed, packaged food!

ON UNSEEN BENEFITS

Michelle Newman, excerpt from "So My Kids Are Picky Eaters. Get Over It" on You're My Favorite Today blog

When my child was six years old, I'd had it with her picky eating. I was sick and tired of having to make a pot of mac and cheese with every meal my husband and I ate just so she'd have something to eat.

I tried tough love. One night, I made lasagna, which she, of course, couldn't even look at without gagging. We put a small square on her plate (no lie, it was like a one-inch square) and told her she had to eat it before she could leave the table. Swear to God, that child sat at the table crying for over two hours with us yelling and threatening and storming around as the clock ticked away. And (spoiler alert) she didn't ever eat the lasagna. If we hadn't changed the consequence (the details of which, all these years later, I have forgotten) she might very well still be sitting at the table today, twelve years later.

I did what most first-time moms do when all else fails. I took her to the doctor, and to this day, I am grateful to that woman for her advice. She told us things we already knew and had tried, things that had been a source of frustration in their failure for years:

- Have your child help plan the meal (done, many, many times, and which always resulted in the same thing: peanut butter and jelly and apple bites).
- Make sure your child knows that it is the parents' job to cook the dinner and the child's job to eat the dinner, and the consequence of refusal is hunger. (Harsh, but okay, I could live with that as long as my child didn't end up looking like a sad, malnourished child that large groups of famous singers were singing songs about).
- Always have at least one thing on the table that your child likes. (In our case, a basket of bread and a bowl of apple bites. Every night).
- Most importantly? Do not make dinnertime a battle.

The doctor told us to go home and recommit ourselves to these rules for two months, however pointless we thought they were, and then return for a follow-up visit. In the next two months, nothing changed. My child still only ate carbs and apples and didn't try one new thing, but my husband and I kept our mouths shut and followed the rules. When we went back to the doctor two months later, she asked us how dinner had been going. At the exact same time, I said "terrible" and she said "great!"

Huh?

The doctor looked at my daughter and asked her why she answered that way, and she said, "Because dinnertime isn't so mean anymore, and I'm not sad at the table."

Here's the lesson in that six-year-old's honest statement (as told to me by the doctor, but that I still carry with me, all these years later): As a parent, don't make food a control issue with your children (this is especially important with girls). Eating shouldn't be associated with stress or fear. Lay out clear expectations and try your best not to cater to your child, but don't make eating be about power on either side of the table.

UNTIL NEXT TIME

My hope is that you have gained a whole new perspective on picky eating and feel inspired about your child's future. May your family table be enjoyable, nourishing, and full of connection.

PUTTING IT ALL TOGETHER

You made it! Below is a summary of *From Picky to Powerful's* key points for your review. Come to this page as a reference when feeding gets challenging. For example, your mindset might gradually shift to distrust and resistance, which affects how you feed (strategy) and your child's reaction. As time goes by, you might need to review The Strategy section to problem solve or the Know-How section for a boost of motivation.

The road to feeding kids can feel overwhelming and dissatisfying at times, but it can also be incredibly rewarding. My wish is that you are able to empower your kids to be the best eaters they can be.

THE MINDSET

- Understand the difference between normal and problematic picky eating.
- Trust your child to do well with eating while accepting his eating capabilities.
- Meet your child where she is knowing this stage, no matter how long, will not last forever.
- Have high expectations for eating without pressure by continually offering foods with an expectant attitude no

matter how many times it is rejected.

The Strategies

- Offer regular meals at predictable times and in a designated area.
- Plan and provide a variety of foods at those meals and snacks, both liked and not yet accepted.
- Eat together as often as possible and serve items family-style so family members can serve themselves.
- Make mealtime pleasant and free from pressure by utilizing Satter's Division of Responsibility.
- Understand how to meet nutritional needs with food and supplements if needed.

The Know-How

- Discover child-friendly ways to offer nutritious foods.
- Take on the role of "food teacher" and spend time educating your child about food without the intention of getting her to eat.
- Take exposure up a notch by encouraging children to explore, prepare, and become independent with food.
- Have faith in the process and reach out to other experienced parents when you need some encouragement.

ABOUT THE AUTHOR

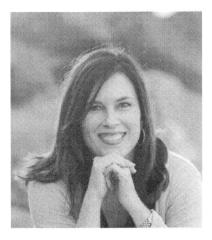

Maryann Jacobsen is a registered dietitian, independent author, and speaker. She is founding editor of Raise Healthy Eaters (now MaryannJacobsen.com) and runs The Healthy Family Podcast. Maryann's books, blog, and podcast aim to revolutionize the health of families through improving their relationship with food. Her writing has appeared in the New York Times, Los Angeles Times, Mindbodygreen, and She Knows. She has been quoted in various publications including *Parents, Scholastic Parent & Child,* and *American Profile* and has been featured on *Good Morning America.* Find out more at MaryannJacobsen.com.

Other titles from Maryann include:

How to Raise a Mindful Eater: 8 Powerful Principles for Transforming Your Child's Relationship with Food: The book pinpoints 8 Powerful Principles that give you the best shot at raising a mindful eater, someone who listens to their body, eats for nourishment and enjoyment, and naturally eats in moderation.

The Family Dinner Solution: How to Create a Rotation of Dinner Meals Your Family Will Love: In a step-by-step format, you'll learn how to create a core rotation of dinner meals that will satisfy even your pickiest family members.

Fearless Feeding: How to Raise Healthy Eaters From High Chair to High School: Considered the bible of feeding kids, you'll get the What, How and Why of feeding at each stage of development — infancy, toddlerhood, school age, adolescence and adulthood. You'll learn what to expect in terms of growth, child development (the why of eating) and how to meet nutritional needs.

What Does Your Tummy Say?: A children's story that highlights the importance of tuning into hunger and fullness. It can serve as a conversation starter for families to share experiences and challenges, and learn about healthy ways to relate to food.

Sign up for Maryann's email list and get her FREE e-book, *The Landmines of a Healthy Relationship with Food.* Go to MaryannJacobsen.com/list.

NOTES

Introduction

1. Cardona Cano, Sebastian, Henning Tiemeier, Daphne Van Hoeken, Anne Tharner, Vincent W. V. Jaddoe, Albert Hofman, Frank C. Verhulst, and Hans W. Hoek. "Trajectories of Picky Eating During Childhood: A General Population Study." *International Journal of Eating Disorders* 48, no. 6 (January 30, 2015): 570–79. doi:10.1002/eat.22384.

2. Kurcinka, Mary Sheedy. *Raising Your Spirited Child: A Guide for Parents Whose Child Is More Intense, Sensitive, Perceptive, Persistent, and Energetic.* New York: William Morrow Paperbacks, 2006.

3. Kessler, Jason. "A Picky Eater Turned Top Chef." October 27, 2011. Accessed November 2, 2016. http://www.foodrepublic.com/2011/10/27/picky-eater-turned-top-chef.

4. Rosenthal, Robert and Lenore Jacobsen. "Teachers Expectancies: Determinants of Pupils' IQ Gains." *Psychological Reports,* 19, no. 1 (August 1966): 115–18. doi:10.2466/pro.1966.19.1.115.

5. Satter, Ellyn. "Division of Responsibility in Feeding." 2016. Accessed October 7, 2016. http://ellynsatterinstitute.org/dor/divisionofresponsibilityinfeeding.php.

Chapter 1

1. Toomey, Kay. "Picky Eaters Vs. Problem Feeders – Dr. Kay Toomey." 2016. Accessed November 2, 2016. http://www.sosapproach-conferences.com/articles/picky-eaters-vs-problem-feeders.

2. Dovey, Terence M., Paul A. Staples, E. Leigh Gibson, and Jason C. G. Halford. "Food Neophobia and 'picky/fussy' Eating in Children: A Review." *Appetite,* 50, no. 2-3 (March 2008): 181–93. doi:10.1016/j.appet.2007.09.009.

3. Cardona Cano, Sebastian, Henning Tiemeier, Daphne Van Hoeken, Anne Tharner, Vincent W. V. Jaddoe, Albert Hofman, Frank C. Verhulst, and Hans W. Hoek. "Trajectories of Picky Eating During Childhood: A General Population Study." *International Journal of Eating Disorders,* 48, no. 6 (January 30, 2015): 570–79. doi:10.1002/eat.22384.

4. AAP Committee on Nutrition and Ronald E. Kleinman MD FAAP. *Pediatric Nutrition Handbook.* 6th ed. American Academy of Pediatrics, 2008.

5. Fisher, JO, JA Mennella, SO Hughes, Y Liu, PM Mendoza, and H Patrick. "Offering 'Dip' Promotes Intake of a Moderately-Liked Raw Vegetable Among Preschoolers with Genetic Sensitivity to Bitterness." *Journal of the Academy of Nutrition and Dietetics,* 112, no. 2 (June 29, 2012): 235–45.

6. Fildes, A, van Jaarsveld, CH Llewellyn, A Fisher, L Cooke, and J Wardle. "Nature and Nurture in Children's Food Preferences." *The American Journal of Clinical Nutrition,* 99, no. 4 (January 31, 2014): 911–17.

7. Satter, Ellyn. *Child of Mine: Feeding with Love and Good Sense.* Revised ed. Boulder, Colorado: Bull Publishing Company, 2000.

8. Committee on Injury, Violence and Poison Prevention. "Prevention of Choking Among Children." *Pediatrics,* 125, no. 3 (February 22, 2010): 601–7. doi:10.1542/peds.2009-2862.

9. Castle, Jill and Maryann Jacobsen. *Fearless Feeding: How to Raise Healthy Eaters from High Chair to High School.* San Francisco: Jossey Bass, 2013.

10. Smith, A. D., A. Fildes, L. Cooke, M. Herle, N. Shakeshaft, R. Plomin, and C. Llewellyn. "Genetic and Environmental Influences on Food Preferences in Adolescence." *American Journal of Clinical Nutrition* 104, no. 2 (July 6, 2016): 446–53. doi:10.3945/ajcn.116.133983.

Chapter 2

1. Toomey, Kay. "Picky Eaters Vs. Problem Feeders – Dr. Kay Toomey." 2016. Accessed November 2, 2016. http://www.sosapproach-conferences.com/articles/picky-eaters-vs-problem-feeders.

2. Toomey, Kay. "Red Flags – Dr. Kay Toomey." 2016. Accessed November 2, 2016. http://www.sosapproach-conferences.com/articles/red-flags.

3. Disorders. "Avoidant Restrictive Food Intake Disorder." 2016. Accessed November 2, 2016. http://www.disorders.org/avoidant-restrictive-food-intake-disorder.

Chapter 3

1. Slaughter, CW and AH Bryant. "Hungry for Love: The Feeding Relationship in the Psychological Development of Young Children." *The Permanente journal,* 8, no. 1 (January 1, 2004): 23–29.

2. Castle, Jill and Maryann Jacobsen. *Fearless Feeding: How to Raise Healthy Eaters from High Chair to High*

School. San Francisco: Jossey Bass, 2013.

3. Satter, Ellyn. "The Feeding Relationship: Problems and Interventions." *The Journal of Pediatrics,* 117, no. 2 (August 1990): S181–89. doi:10.1016/s0022-3476(05)80017-4.

Chapter 4

1. Isacco, L., N. Lazaar, S. Ratel, D. Thivel, J. Aucouturier, E. Doré, M. Meyer, and P. Duché. "The Impact of Eating Habits on Anthropometric Characteristics in French Primary School Children." *Child: Care, Health and Development,* 36, no. 6 (July 14, 2010): 835–42. doi:10.1111/j.1365-2214.2010.01113.x.

2. AAP Committee on Nutrition and Ronald E. Kleinman MD FAAP. *Pediatric Nutrition Handbook.* 6th ed. American Academy of Pediatrics, 2008.

3. Hammons, A. J. and B. H. Fiese. "Is Frequency of Shared Family Meals Related to the Nutritional Health of Children and Adolescents?" *Pediatrics,* 127, no. 6 (May 2, 2011): e1565–e1574. doi:10.1542/peds.2010-1440.

4. Tanofsky-Kraff, M, H.L. Hyanos, L.A. Kotler LA, and J.A. Yanovski. "Laboratory-Based Studies of Eating Among Children and Adolescents." *Current Nutrition & Food Science,* 3, no. 1 (February 1, 2007): 55–74. doi:10.2174/1573401310703010055.

5. Satter, Ellyn. *Child of Mine: Feeding with Love and Good Sense.* Revised ed. Boulder, Colorado: Bull Publishing Company, 2000.

Chapter 5

1. Blissett, Jackie, Carmel Bennett, Anna Fogel, Gillian Harris, and Suzanne Higgs. "Parental Modelling and Prompting Effects on Acceptance of a Novel Fruit in 2–4-Year-Old Children Are Dependent on Children's

Food Responsiveness." *British Journal of Nutrition,* 115, no. 03 (November 25, 2015): 554–64. doi:10.1017/s0007114515004651.

2. Satter, Ellyn. "Division of Responsibility in Feeding." 2016. Accessed October 7, 2016. http://ellynsatterinstitute.org/dor/divisionofresponsibilityinfeeding.php.

3. Orrell-Valente, Joan K., Laura G. Hill, Whitney A. Brechwald, Kenneth A. Dodge, Gregory S. Pettit, and John E. Bates. "'Just three more bites': An Observational Analysis of Parents' Socialization of Children's Eating at Mealtime." *Appetite,* 48, no. 1 (January 2007): 37–45. doi:10.1016/j.appet.2006.06.006.

4. Loth, K. A., R. F. MacLehose, J. A. Fulkerson, S. Crow, and D. Neumark-Sztainer. "Food-Related Parenting Practices and Adolescent Weight Status: A Population-Based Study." *Pediatrics,* 131, no. 5 (April 22, 2013): e1443–e1450. doi:10.1542/peds.2012-3073.

5. Galloway, Amy T., Laura M. Fiorito, Lori A. Francis, and Leann L. Birch. "'Finish Your Soup': Counterproductive Effects of Pressuring Children to Eat on Intake and Affect." *Appetite,* 46, no. 3 (May 2006): 318–23. doi:10.1016/j.appet.2006.01.019.

6. Cooke, Lucy J., Lucy C. Chambers, Elizabeth V. Añez, and Jane Wardle. "Facilitating or Undermining? The Effect of Reward on Food Acceptance. A Narrative Review." *Appetite,* 57, no. 2 (October 2011): 493–97. doi:10.1016/j.appet.2011.06.016.

7. Fildes, Alison, Cornelia H. M. van Jaarsveld, Jane Wardle, and Lucy Cooke. "Parent-Administered Exposure to Increase Children's Vegetable Acceptance: A Randomized Controlled Trial." *Journal of the Academy of Nutrition and Dietetics,* 114, no. 6 (June 2014): 881–88. doi:10.1016/j.jand.2013.07.040.

8. Remington, A., E. Annez, H. Croker, J. Wardle, and L. Cooke. "Increasing Food Acceptance in the Home Setting: A Randomized Controlled Trial of Parent-Administered Taste Exposure with Incentives." *American Journal of Clinical Nutrition,* 95, no. 1 (December 7, 2011): 72–77. doi:10.3945/ajcn.111.024596.

9. Añez, E., A. Remington, J. Wardle, and L. Cooke. "The Impact of Instrumental Feeding on Children's Responses to Taste Exposure." *Journal of Human Nutrition and Dietetics,* 26, no. 5 (December 17, 2012): 415–20. doi:10.1111/jhn.12028.

10. Just, David R. and Joseph Price. "Using Incentives to Encourage Healthy Eating in Children." *Journal of Human Resources,* 48, no. 4 (2013): 855–72. doi:10.1353/jhr.2013.0029.

11. Upton, Dominic, Penney Upton, and Charlotte Taylor. "Increasing Children's Lunchtime Consumption of Fruit and Vegetables: An Evaluation of the Food Dudes Programme." *Public Health Nutrition,* 16, no. 06 (October 16, 2012): 1066–72. doi:10.1017/s1368980012004612.

12. Deci, E.L., R. Koestner, and R.M. Ryan. "A Meta-Analytic Review of Experiments Examining the Effects of Extrinsic Rewards on Intrinsic Motivation." *Psychological Bulletin,* 125, no. 6 (1999): 627–68. doi:10.1037//0033-2909.125.6.627.

13. Cameron, J, KM Banko, and WD Pierce. "Pervasive Negative Effects of Rewards on Intrinsic Motivation: The Myth Continues." *The Behavior Analyst.* 24, no. 1 (April 1, 2001): 1–44.

14. Kohn, Alfie. "The Risks of Rewards." December 3, 1994. Accessed November 2, 2016. http://www.alfiekohn.org/teaching/ror.htm.

15. Leford, Gerard E., Meiyu Fang, and Berry Gerhart.

"Negative Effects of Extrinsic Rewards on Intrinsic Motivation: More Smoke Than Fire." February 2013. Accessed November 2, 2016. https://ceo.usc.edu/negative-effects-of-extrinsic-rewards-on-intrinsic-motivation-more-smoke-than-fire/.

Chapter 6

1. Bailey, Regan L., Victor L. Fulgoni, Debra R. Keast, Cindy V. Lentino, and Johanna T. Dwyer. "Do Dietary Supplements Improve Micronutrient Sufficiency in Children and Adolescents?" *The Journal of Pediatrics,* 161, no. 5 (November 2012): 837–42.e3. doi:10.1016/j.jpeds.2012.05.009.

2. AAP Committee on Nutrition and Ronald E. Kleinman MD FAAP. *Pediatric Nutrition Handbook.* 6th ed. American Academy of Pediatrics, 2008.

3. Burlingame, Barbara, Chizuru Nishida, Ricardo Uauy, and Robert Weisell. "Fats and Fatty Acids in Human Nutrition: Introduction." *Annals of Nutrition and Metabolism,* 55, no. 1-3 (2009): 5–7. doi:10.1159/000228993.

4. Wagner, C. L. and F. R. Greer. "Prevention of Rickets and Vitamin D Deficiency in Infants, Children, and Adolescents." *Pediatrics,* 122, no. 5 (October 31, 2008): 1142–52. doi:10.1542/peds.2008-1862.

Chapter 7

1. Fisher, JO, JA Mennella, SO Hughes, Y Liu, PM Mendoza, and H Patrick. "Offering 'Dip' Promotes Intake of a Moderately-Liked Raw Vegetable Among Preschoolers with Genetic Sensitivity to Bitterness." *Journal of the Academy of Nutrition and Dietetics.* 112, no. 2 (June 29, 2012): 235–45.

2. Billon, Karen Le. *French Kids Eat Everything: How*

Our Family Moved to France, Cured Picky Eating, Banished Snacking, and Discovered 10 Simple Rules for Raising Healthy, Happy Eaters. New York: HarperCollins Publishers, 2012.

3. Zeinstra, G. G., C. de Graaf, and M. A. Koelen. "The Influence of Preparation Method on Children's Liking for Vegetables." *Appetite,* 51, no. 3 (November 2008): 757. doi:10.1016/j.appet.2008.05.028.

4. Spill, M. K., L. L. Birch, L. S. Roe, and B. J. Rolls. "Eating Vegetables First: The Use of Portion Size to Increase Vegetable Intake in Preschool Children." *American Journal of Clinical Nutrition,* 91, no. 5 (March 10, 2010): 1237–43. doi:10.3945/ajcn.2009.29139.

5. Butte, Nancy F., Mary Kay Fox, Ronette R. Briefel, Anna Maria Siega-Riz, Johanna T. Dwyer, Denise M. Deming, and Kathleen C. Reidy. "Nutrient Intakes of US Infants, Toddlers, and Preschoolers Meet or Exceed Dietary Reference Intakes." *Journal of the American Dietetic Association,* 110, no. 12 (December 2010): S27–S37. doi:10.1016/j.jada.2010.09.004.

6. Niinikoski, H., K. Pahkala, M. Ala-Korpela, J. Viikari, T. Ronnemaa, H. Lagstrom, E. Jokinen, et al. "Effect of Repeated Dietary Counseling on Serum Lipoproteins from Infancy to Adulthood." *Pediatrics,* 129, no. 3 (February 13, 2012): e704–13. doi:10.1542/peds.2011-1503.

Chapter 8

1. Van der Horst, Klazine, Aurore Ferrage, and Andreas Rytz. "Involving Children in Meal Preparation. Effects on Food Intake." *Appetite,* 79 (August 2014): 18–24. doi:10.1016/j.appet.2014.03.030.

2. Lythcott-Haimes, Julie. *How to Raise an Adult: Break Free of the Overparenting Trap and Prepare Your Kid.*

St. Martin's Griffin: New York, 2016.

Chapter 9

1. Sampson, Sally and Natalie Digate Muth. "Can Young Picky Eaters Reform? 10 Rules, and a Plan." *New York Times Well Family*, September 16, 2015. Accessed on December 15, 2016. http://parenting.blogs.nytimes.com/2015/09/16/can-young-picky-eaters-reform-10-rules-and-a-plan/

2. Brown-Worsham, Sasha. "An Open Letter to the Moms Who Judged My Kids for Being Picky Eaters." Yahoo Parenting, April 3, 2015. Accessed December 15, 2016. https://www.yahoo.com/news/an-open-letter-to-the-moms-who-judged-my-kids-for-115349417407.html.

3. Fildes, A, van Jaarsveld, CH Llewellyn, A Fisher, L Cooke, and J Wardle. "Nature and Nurture in Children's Food Preferences." *The American Journal of Clinical Nutrition*. 99, no. 4 (January 31, 2014): 911–17.

4. Dovey, Terence M., Paul A. Staples, E. Leigh Gibson, and Jason C. G. Halford. "Food Neophobia and 'picky/fussy' Eating in Children: A Review." *Appetite*, 50, no. 2-3 (March 2008): 181–93. doi:10.1016/j.appet.2007.09.009.

5. Grummer-Strawn, L. M., R. Li, C. G. Perrine, K. S. Scanlon, and S. B. Fein. "Infant Feeding and Long-Term Outcomes: Results from the Year 6 Follow-up of Children in the Infant Feeding Practices Study II." *Pediatrics*, 134, no. Supplement (September 1, 2014): S1–S3. doi:10.1542/peds.2014-0646b.

6. US Department of Health and Human Services; US Department of Agriculture. *2015-2020 Dietary Guidelines for Americans*. 8th ed. Washington, DC: US Dept of Health and Human Services; December 2015. http://www.health.gov/DietaryGuidelines.

Accessed March 14, 2016.

7. Lahey, Jessica. *The Gift of Failure: How the Best Parents Learn to Let Go So Their Children Can Succeed.* Harper Paperbacks; Reprint edition: New York, 2016.

8. Van Zetten, Skye. "Beef and a Pancake." January 16, 2015. Accessed November 2, 2016. https://mealtimehostage.com/2015/01/15/beef-and-a-pancake/.

9. Remmer, Sarah. "The Game-Changing Question Parents of Picky Eaters Need to Ask." January 1, 2016. Accessed November 2, 2016. http://www.sarahremmer.com/the-game-changing-question-that-parents-of-picky-eaters-need-to-ask/.

10. Roskelley, Amy. "Scrumptious Blueberry Salad." Accessed November 2, 2016. http://www.superhealthykids.com/scrumptious-blueberry-salad/.

Printed in Great Britain
by Amazon